Empowering Social Workers

Manohar Pawar · Richard Hugman
Andrew Alexandra · A.W. (Bill) Anscombe
Editors

Empowering Social Workers

Virtuous Practitioners

Springer

Editors
Manohar Pawar
School of Humanities and Social Sciences
Charles Sturt University
Wagga Wagga, NSW
Australia

Andrew Alexandra
Department of Philosophy
The University of Melbourne
Parkville, VIC
Australia

Richard Hugman
School of Social Sciences
University of New South Wales
Sydney, NSW
Australia

A.W. (Bill) Anscombe
School of Humanities and Social Sciences
Charles Sturt University
Wagga Wagga, NSW
Australia

ISBN 978-981-10-3808-2 ISBN 978-981-10-3809-9 (eBook)
DOI 10.1007/978-981-10-3809-9

Library of Congress Control Number: 2017930406

Printed on acid-free paper

This Springer imprint is published by Springer Nature
The registered company is Springer Nature Singapore Pte Ltd.
The registered company address is: 152 Beach Road, #21-01/04 Gateway East, Singapore 189721, Singapore

Acknowledgements

We have greatly enjoyed researching social workers' practice and have learned a good deal from the insightful and inspiring life stories, qualities and practice wisdom of the practitioners presented in this book. For frankly sharing their personal and professional life experiences, we immensely thank ten social workers who kindly agreed to participate in the project, which required long and demanding interviews. We specially invited six colleagues, whose names appear at the head of their respective chapters, to join us in conducting interviews and co-authoring chapters with us, and we really appreciate their time for this research project.

In addition to all authors, we invited Prof. Tom Campbell, Prof. Mel Gray, Dr. Graeme McLean, Dr. Rose Melville and Mr. Arif Rehman to participate in a two-day workshop to thoroughly discuss each chapter and, based on that high quality discussion, the writing was further refined. We are grateful for their generosity in providing their time and thoughts. We also thank Ms. Narrelle Ingold for her outstanding assistance in organising the workshop and Ms. Nikki Scott and Ms. Debra Noy from the Institute for Land, Water and Society for providing excellent administrative assistance. We thank Ms. Heather Kelly for editing the final manuscript.

This research was supported under the Australian Research Council's Discovery Project funding scheme (DP140103730; project title, *Virtuous Practitioners: Empowering Social Workers*) and we are grateful to all those who have offered comments and suggestions on the grant application, and contributed to this decision. We are also grateful to Charles Sturt University's Human Research Ethics Committee for approving the research proposal (protocol no: 2014/057).

We would also like to thank peer reviewers of the book proposal. At Springer, we greatly appreciate the work of Ms. Ilaria Walker, Mr. Nick Melchior and their team in facilitating the commissioning process and their commitment to publishing it. Thanks also to Roman Mr. Ashok Kadam for his efficient copy editing and to Mr. Henry Pravin Arokiaraj for successfully managing the production of the book in a professional and friendly manner.

In essence, this book is a product of excellent teamwork. However, for any shortcomings and limitations in it, we are responsible.

Manohar Pawar
Richard Hugman
Andrew Alexandra
A.W. (Bill) Anscombe

Contents

1 **Introduction—The Role of Virtues in Social Work Practice** 1
Manohar Pawar, Richard Hugman, Andrew Alexandra and A.W. (Bill) Anscombe

2 **Voice to the Voiceless—Sue Ash, AO** 17
Christina Fernandes and Richard Hugman

3 **But You Can Push and Push and Push—Diana Batzias** 37
Manohar Pawar

4 **Empower People to Take Control of Their Own Lives—Tom Calma, AO** 53
Andrew Alexandra and Manohar Pawar

5 **Respect and Integrity—John Gavaghan** 77
A.W. (Bill) Anscombe and Emma Rush

6 **What Can We Do to Make Changes?—Virginia (Ginni) Hall, AO** 87
Emma Rush and A.W. (Bill) Anscombe

7 **A People World, Rather Than a Paper World—Bronwyn Hyde** 101
Manohar Pawar and Wendy Bowles

8 **I Cannot Give up, I Cannot Give up on the Children—Bernadette McMenamin, AO** 123
Manohar Pawar and Linda Briskman

9 **You Roll up Your Sleeves and You Help, and Work with People—Robyn Miller** 139
Manohar Pawar and Sharlene Nipperess

10 Hunger for Movement and Action—Sue Vardon, AO 157
Manohar Pawar and Sue King

11 What You Know Plays Out in Action—Jill Wilson, AO 179
A.W. (Bill) Anscombe

12 Virtue-Led Social Work Practice 193
Manohar Pawar, Richard Hugman, Andrew Alexandra
and A.W. (Bill) Anscombe

Editors and Contributors

About the Editors

Manohar Pawar is Professor of Social Work at the School of Humanities and Social Sciences, Charles Sturt University and is the President of the Asia-Pacific branch of the International Consortium for Social Development. He has over 30 years of experience in social work education, research and practice in Australia and India. He is the lead chief investigator of research funded by the Australian Research Council's Discovery project that focuses on virtues and social work practice. Manohar has received a number of awards, including Citation Award for Outstanding Contributions to Student Learning (2008, from the Australian Learning and Teaching Council); and Quality of Life Award (2001, from the Association of Commonwealth Universities). His interests and recent publications include *Future Directions in Social Development* (Palgrave Macmillan 2017); *Reflective Social Work Practice: Thinking, doing and being* (Cambridge University Press 2015); *Water and Social Policy* (Palgrave Macmillan 2014); *Social and Community Development Practice* (Sage 2014); *International Social Work: Issues, strategies and programs* (2nd edition, Sage 2013); and *Sage Handbook of International Social Work* (Ed., Sage 2012).

Richard Hugman is currently Professor of Social Work at the University of New South Wales and has practised, taught and researched in Australia and the United Kingdom. From 2002 to 2008, he was a member of the International Federation of Social Workers ethics committee and subsequently chaired the committee from 2008 to 2014. Richard has published widely on ethics, including *Rethinking Values and Ethics in Social Work* (Palgrave Macmillan 2016); *Culture, Values and Ethics in Social Work: Embracing diversity* (Routledge 2013); *New Approaches for Ethics for the Caring Professions* (Palgrave Macmillan 2005).

Andrew Alexandra is Senior Research Fellow in the Australian Research Council Special Research Centre for Applied Philosophy and Public Ethics at the University of Melbourne, with research and teaching interests in political philosophy and professional and applied ethics. Among his many publications in these areas are his co-authored books *Reason, Values and Institutions* (Tertiary Press 2002), *Police Ethics* (Allen & Unwin 2nd edition 2006), *Ethics in Practice: Moral theory and the professions* (UNSW Press 2009), *Integrity Systems for Occupations* (Ashgate 2010), and *Media, Markets, and Morcals* (Wiley-Blackwell 2011), and his co-edited book, *Private Military and Security Companies: Ethics, policies and civil-military relations* (Routledge 2008). Andrew has engaged in consultancies and collaborative research projects with a range of professional groups, including the Australian Association of Social Workers, Victoria Police, the Safety Institute of Australia, the Consumers Health Forum, the Professional Standards Council (New South Wales) and the Australian Anthropological Society.

A.W. (Bill) Anscombe is Adjunct Associate Professor of Social Work at Charles Sturt University (CSU). Prior to retiring, he had 21 years at CSU and before that 20 years in Corrections, where he held trainee to senior management positions. He was seconded from the university to be the Director for Child Protection (Western) as part of the then New South Wales Department of Community Services, with responsibility for 70% of the state geographically. He also operated in a joint appointment between CSU and the Department of Community Services for 4 years. He is currently a voluntary director of four not-for-profit small/medium human service companies or associations. He has an active, committed Christian faith. Bill's research interests and projects have been broad, including in the areas of Indigenous housing and governance, multicultural Australia, rural social services and numerous service evaluations. His doctoral studies were on "Consilience in social work: Reflections on thinking, doing and being". His most recent publication is *Reflective Social Work Practice: Thinking, doing and being* (Cambridge University Press 2015).

Contributors

Wendy Bowles is Professor of Social Work and Human Services at Charles Sturt University and Acting Head of School of Humanities and Social Sciences. Wendy's main practice area and her Ph.D. research are in the disability field and professional practice, working from citizenship and relational perspectives. Her teaching and research interests also include professional practice, ethics, eco-social work, field education and rural practice. Wendy is co-author of two books: *Research for Social Workers: An introduction to methods* (3rd edition, Allen & Unwin 2012) and *Ethical Practice in Social Work* (Allen & Unwin 2006). She has published numerous book chapters and refereed journal papers, enjoys working with and supervising research students and practitioners, and has participated in several national research projects into field education, which have produced online resources for practitioners, students and academics.

Linda Briskman is Professor in Margaret Whitlam Chair of Social Work at Western Sydney University. Her main areas of research and activism are Indigenous rights, asylum seeker rights and countering Islamophobia. She has an interest in bioethics, including collaborative projects on the health of Afghans in Iran and ethical issues related to health and welfare professionals employed in immigration detention settings. Linda extensively publishes her research. Her most recent book is *Social Work with Indigenous Communities: A human rights approach* (The Federation Press 2014). She also engages regularly in media commentary and opinion pieces, and plays a lead role in change-focused networks, including Voices Against Bigotry, Social Workers Without Borders and Academics for Refugees.

Christina Fernandes is a lecturer and course co-ordinator in the Department of Social Work, in the School of Occupational Therapy and Social Work at Curtin University. Tina's Ph.D. explored the relationality inherent in work between social workers and language interpreters in torture and trauma services. Her research interests are in the areas of homelessness and substance use, the service and support needs of carers (mothers, parents and grandparents) and the lived experiences of mothers with children with disabilities. Tina has recently completed an industry-funded research project that sought to work using the principles and processes of coproduction.

Sue King is a social worker and former Discipline Head, Social Work and Human Services at the University of South Australia. Her current roles are in the field of organisational governance. She is Chair of Uniting Communities Inc. and a board member of several other not-for-profit organisations. Sue is an active member of the Australian Association of Social Workers and a past president of the South Australian branch. As a member of the University of South Australia Centre for Social Change, Sue's research and writing focuses on the impact of social policy on the delivery of human services, the governance of human service organisations and the conceptualisation of workers.

Sharlene Nipperess is a lecturer in social work at RMIT University. Her research focuses on critical human rights based practice, social work ethics, critical multicultural practice, green social work, and practice with refugees and asylum seekers and people experiencing mental distress. She is concerned with exploring the relationship between these issues and the implications for social work education. Sharlene is President of Australia and New Zealand Social Work and Welfare Education and Research (ANZSWWER). Her most recent publication is *Doing Critical Social Work: Transformative practices for social justice* (co-edited, Allen & Unwin 2016).

Emma Rush is a lecturer in philosophy and ethics at the School of Humanities and Social Sciences and a member of the Centre for Applied Philosophy and Public Ethics at Charles Sturt University. She teaches professional ethics to human services, health and creative industries students, as well as history of philosophy subjects. She is nationally recognised for her research on the sexualisation of children. She was the lead author of two papers on this subject released by the Australia Institute in 2006. These papers prompted considerable public debate, ultimately leading to a Senate Inquiry into the issue. Emma continues to write and speak about the sexualisation of children to academic, professional and general audiences. Within applied ethics, Emma's other major research areas are professional ethics and environmental ethics.

Chapter 1
Introduction—The Role of Virtues in Social Work Practice

Manohar Pawar, Richard Hugman, Andrew Alexandra and A.W. (Bill) Anscombe

This book presents ten short biographies of professional social workers who have made significant contributions to the wellbeing of individuals, families and communities, and to the effective functioning of government and non-government organisations. The biographies, and associated discussions, aim to help the reader to see the inspiring qualities of character—the virtues—which have helped these social workers to achieve what they have.

The main purpose of this introductory chapter is to explain how we understand the nature of virtue and why we see it as important in social work practice. Virtuous action, as we understand it, is action that is appropriate to the situation that confronts a social worker. Hence, we also provide a brief outline of the socio-economic and political contexts in which the subjects of these biographies worked. We explain, too, how the subjects of the biographies were chosen, and the methods (and their limitations) used to develop their biographies. Finally, we provide a very brief summary of the order and content of the biographies.

M. Pawar (✉) · A.W. (Bill) Anscombe
Charles Sturt University, Wagga Wagga, Australia
e-mail: mpawar@csu.edu.au

A.W. (Bill) Anscombe
e-mail: BAnscombe@csu.edu.au

R. Hugman
University of New South Wales, Sydney, Australia
e-mail: r.hugman@unsw.edu.au

A. Alexandra
University of Melbourne, Melbourne, Australia
e-mail: a.alexandra@unimelb.edu.au

M. Pawar et al. (eds.), *Empowering Social Workers*,
DOI 10.1007/978-981-10-3809-9_1

Meaning of Virtue

The term "virtue" has a range of uses, not all of which bear any moral implications. As our research interactions with social workers suggested that they appreciated the clarity of the concept of virtue at the beginning, and they tended to think of social work values as virtues, and this book is about virtues of a professional practitioner —social worker—it is important to clarify the complex and confusing meaning of virtue at the outset. In simple words, what we mean by virtues is qualities, character, good habits or attributes of practitioners that help them to achieve excellence in their practice. The noun "virtuoso" (Hornby 1992) means a person who is exceptionally or proficiently skilled in the use of knowledge, principles, qualities or attributes and techniques in his or her practice.

The way social workers narrated their professional practice life stories presented in this book indicated that their virtues or qualities invariably combined social work values and principles—certain attributes, roles and functions—often in an overlapping manner. How people internalise certain qualities, develop them and stick to them in the overall social and professional socialisation is a complex process and our conceptualisation may not be able to capture that process and put it into practice. Drawing from the biographic narratives, we have attempted to conceptualise virtue in terms of principles and values, qualities or attributes, and roles and functions, as shown in Fig. 1.1, though they overlap and are inextricably interlinked.

Virtues as Values and Principles

Any person's firm belief in certain values and principles and reflection of those values and principles in words and deeds constitutes a significant part of the virtue in professional practice. For example, social workers' references to action about social justice, anti-discrimination, equality, human rights, gender sensitivity and so on constitute fundamental bases of their virtue, which in turn influence their qualities and attributes and roles and functions to achieve excellence in their own ways.

Fig. 1.1 Delineation of the concept of virtue in social work practice

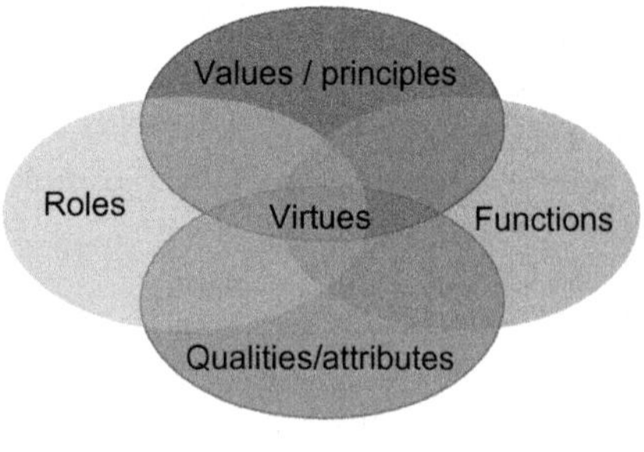

Virtues as Character/Qualities/Attributes

In the virtue ethics tradition stemming from Aristotle, it is held that people aim at a state of flourishing: the virtues are both partially constitutive of that state (as types of excellence), and necessary means to its realisation. Aristotle also saw virtues as a mid-point between vices (MacIntyre 1998, pp. 62–4). For example, the virtue of generosity is the mid-point between meanness and extravagance. Virtues (and vices) are aspects of people's character. A virtue consists of a stable disposition to respond to the world in a certain desirable way. That disposition is multi-faceted—it issues in actions, but it also consists of perceptions, emotions, motivations, desires, judgements and preferences. A generous person is not just one who treats others kindly, but also someone who perceives their needs and is moved by them, feels upset by others' meanness and gladdened by their kindness, prefers the company of other generous people, and so on. The generous person, then, does not simply act kindly—they do so because they perceive that it is the right thing to do and because they find it attractive to do so.

The range, complexity and continually changing nature of the sorts of situations where we may have to act morally, and the idiosyncrasies of the individuals we deal with in those situations, mean that it is impossible to come up with more than very general prescriptions for virtuous action. Freely giving or serving someone what they want will not always count as acting virtuously; for example, sometimes it is better for people not to get what they want—sometimes more good will be done by giving the things that someone wants to others, or keeping it for oneself. Hence, the exercise of virtue requires good judgement. The ability to make accurate judgements about how to act in particular circumstances is what Aristotle calls practical wisdom (*phronesis*). Hence practical wisdom is a kind of master virtue; it is only those who possess practical wisdom who can be counted as virtuous. Practical wisdom is an achievement, the product of experience and instruction. As Aristotle famously said, "Neither by nature nor contrary to nature do the virtues arise in us; rather we are adapted by nature to receive them, and are made perfect by habit". Many of the events in the working lives of the social workers described in this book demonstrate the exercise of practical wisdom—and in some cases, the painful process of gaining it.

Virtues as Roles and Functions

Generally, as functions emanate from roles and sometimes a dominant function can be considered as a role (for example, counsellor as the role and counselling as a major function that requires many other functions along with values or principles and qualities to achieve excellence), roles and functions are discussed together to clarify and develop the concept of virtue as presented in Fig. 1.1. Often roles are embedded in positions as social worker, counsellor, community development officer, director/administrator/manager, senior clinical social worker, supervisor and so on. As an example, one important function of all these roles is listening: listening well with empathy, attentiveness, compassion and readiness to act appropriately, if needed, is a virtue, and pretending to listen without any of these may be considered a vice. Sometimes functions can be ends, as in some cases what people need is a good listener.

This point may be well made by drawing an example from artefacts. Obviously, artefacts have ends in the sense of functions (indeed they are defined by their function); it is not obvious that people do. For instance, we can talk about the virtues of a knife, which include sharpness and ease of handling, or the virtues of a clock, such as accuracy and quietness. Given that sharpness counts as a virtue in a knife, but not in a clock, what do these features of things have in common, such that they all can be called virtues? Each of them counts as a virtue because it helps the object in which it is found to achieve its function. The function of a knife is to cut: being sharp allows the knife to cut, so sharpness is a virtue in a knife. The function of a clock is to keep time: accuracy is necessary for it to be able to keep time, so accuracy is a virtue in a clock. Another way of talking about functions in this sense is to speak of ends: the end for which a knife is intended is cutting, and so on. In general, a virtue can be characterised as some property, the possession of which helps a thing achieve its end.

Artefacts clearly have functions, which define them. Similarly, so do occupational roles, some of which are stated above. To clarify: the function of a doctor is to cure the sick, that of a comedian is to make us laugh. Role virtues are those qualities that help role occupants achieve their function (and role vices are those qualities that get in the way of achieving it). Some virtues—such as listening, diligence and competence—seem relevant to all occupational roles, though their specific form may vary from role to role. But others are relativised to particular roles, or at least take on specific form in different roles. So, manual dexterity is a virtue for a surgeon, but not for a schoolteacher; physical courage is a virtue for a soldier, but not for a clerk; awareness raising and organising people to protest against unjust systems is a virtue for a social worker, but not for a bureaucrat. In some cases a characteristic that counts as a virtue in a role would be seen as a vice in ordinary life or in other roles: suspiciousness is a virtue in a detective, but not in a spouse. In other cases, role virtues are developments of virtues in ordinary morality: respect for autonomy is something we all should have, but may be more central and require more care and thought in some roles, such as that of the social worker.

The relationship between our roles and the rest of our life is complex. For most people, work is of central importance in their life. How well or badly it goes is a central component of the overall experience and assessment of their life. At the same time, work can be an arena in which our inherent aptitudes and reflectively endorsed values can find expression and development; or it can be the place where people indulge their neuroses: to dominate others or to seek approval, say. A reflective practitioner will be conscious of how their personal psychological needs and drives impact on their working life, and in turn on the way their work affects them. To determine what the virtues appropriate to a particular role are, then, we must be clear about the function(s) of that role; and to achieve such roles and functions with excellence, we must be clear about what values or principles and qualities are necessary.

Thus for the purpose of this text, virtues are an integration of values or principles, qualities or attributes, roles and functions of a social worker in a broad sense. In other words, virtues are a relative mix of values, roles and functions buttressed by certain qualities and attributes that are consistently—in tangible and intangible ways—expressed and observed through actions and inactions in terms of emotions, words, deeds, outputs and outcomes. With this conceptual understanding of virtues, now, it may be apt to introduce the rationale of this book.

Background and Rationale of the Book

Social work practice is often conceptualised in terms of "thinking", "doing" and "being/self". "Thinking" refers to the theoretical knowledge base of social work in terms of a range of theories drawn from various social sciences (see Payne 2005; Healy 2005; Gray and Webb 2009; Howe 2009; Cox and Pawar 2013; Teater 2010) and "doing" connotes what social workers do or practise in terms of practice methods, roles and skills (Anscombe 2009; Healy 2012; Hepworth et al. 2002, p. 27; Mowbray 1996; Egan 2010). Crucial to social workers' thinking and doing is their "being/self", which drives the connection between thinking and doing, and directs practice. Although "being/self" of a social worker is the main driver of thinking and doing, the social work profession's education, practice and research have generally been dominated by theory and practice, and practice, and theory in a binary form to the neglect of "being/self".

Although "being/self" of a social worker is all encompassing, comprehensive and may be understood in terms of physiological/organic, mental/emotional, social/relational and spiritual/existential dimensions (see Anscombe 2009; Pawar and Anscombe 2015), for the purpose of our research and this book, with a specific focus, we narrowly treat "being/self" in terms of virtues, qualities or character of social workers (Anscombe 2009). Social work practice historically was born out of some core virtues and values, including compassion, love, commitment, prudence, human dignity and worth, and a critical sense of social justice. Over a hundred years of professionalised practice, particularly under the influence of neo-liberal and market policies, and modern work pressures, we wonder whether the social work profession and practice has moved away from and/or diluted its core values or virtues. Even if it has not, we believe it is vital to strengthen certain qualities and virtues as an integral part of social workers' being/self to serve people better.

Some aspects of current social work education, training and practice, particularly through its code of ethics, appear to suggest that they are heavily tilted towards rules, norms, regulations, procedures, routines, outputs (rather than outcomes) and performance indicators under the dominance of deontological (Kant 1964; Hugman 2005; Banks 2008, 2012; Webb 2010) and consequential/utilitarian (Bowles et al.

2006, p. 61; Furrow 2005, p. 45) traditions, to the extent that often "human being/self" is taken out of practice. Focusing on virtue, quality and character aspects of social worker's being/self, can help to correct that tilt (Aristotle 1976; Hugman and Smith 1995; Clark 2000, 2006; McBeath and Webb 2002, p. 1020; Hugman 2005; Banks 2012; Bowles et al. 2006; Miller 2014).

Further, the social change and social development agenda of the social work profession and unpredictable and uncertain nature of social work practice call for such a focus on social workers' virtues as part of their "being/self". Often the social/structural change/transformation agenda calls for looking beyond rule-bound traditions, though with due respect to them.

> Doing the right thing in social work is not a matter of applying a moral rule, it is not the work-as-activity that is morally right, but rather the worker-as-agent expressed in the range, and subtlety of use, of the virtues. In this sense the virtues are not specific moral concepts, but generalizable capacities of self, the application of which are acquired via training and experience, as described by Aristotle. The morality of the agent comes from his disposition to do the best he can in the circumstances conjoined to good judgement and perception (McBeath and Webb 2002, p. 1026; see also Alexandra and Miller 2009, pp. 65–68; Alexandra and Miller 2010; Annas 2011).

Most importantly, as several social work educators and ethicists have indicated, the virtues have received insufficient consideration in social work theory (Houston 2003; Gray 2010; Pullen-Sansfacon 2010). Despite its significance, the literature shows that social workers' "self" is peripherally referred to, inadequately researched, underdeveloped and underutilised. In addition, social workers' "being/self" is often discussed in the therapeutic context (Coady and Wolgien 1996; Edwards and Bess 1998; Elliott 2000; Reupert 2006) and community development contexts have been largely ignored. Except for theoretical discussions in texts and journal articles (Clark 2000, 2006; Bowles et al. 2006; Hugman 2005; Banks 2008; McBeath and Webb 2002; Webb 2010), to date the use of virtues in social workers' practice has been largely underexplored.

Clark (2006, p. 86) argues that the professional's moral character is relevant to the specific qualities they will bring to their professional role as their character and values will be transmitted in the services and relationships they offer to clients. Further, Clark (2006, pp. 85–86) points out that:

> There is a perpetual tension between the abstract requirements of universal liberal rights and the specific readings of them to be discovered and created in particular contexts. This tension cannot be resolved by reading off from the texts of professional ethics; it must be squarely faced in the everyday judgements made by practising professionals.

McBeath and Webb (2002, p. 1033) suggest that:

> The virtuous worker must learn to bring together strength of mind, judgement, perception of situation and action in a highly analytical way, sorting through alternative courses of action as competing expressions of the good life—of eudaimonia; and these are capacities which have been much discounted by the dilution of the demands of social work training …

Thus they recommend that the profession "develop means by which professionals nurture virtues (p. 1016). This book is one of the means to addressing this important recommendation.

Role of Virtues and Virtue Ethics in Social Work Practice

Virtues in social work practice can be seen as both "formative" and "summative". They are formative in the sense that the development of good social work practice involves the practitioner in learning and refining relevant virtues over a period of time. While some of the appropriate virtues may be present already in the character of the social worker—through prior experience and learning—other aspects of virtue are gained in the process of becoming and being a social worker. In this sense, we can speak of some social workers having "innate" or "natural" personal qualities that appear to suit them well to their professional role. Others can be regarded as having learned well in the processes of education and training, both on formal university programs and through the practice in which they are engaged. The question is not whether social workers are "born or made", but rather how any particular practitioner can build on the combination of their innate character and continual learning opportunities to forge practice that service users, colleagues and they themselves can regard as "good".

In their detailed analysis of virtues in social work and health care, Banks and Gallagher (2009) identify seven particular virtues of practice. These, they argue, are wisdom, care, respectfulness, trustworthiness, justice, courage and integrity. For example, the wise practitioner does not simply take information at face value, but is able to weigh it against past experience to form judgements about how to act that respond to the nuances of a situation. Similarly, the courageous practitioner is one who is able to maintain a commitment to pursue good objectives when to do so is demanding (of energy, time and focus). Courage is not only demonstrated against overt opposition, although that is when it is most clearly evident to many people. In a world in which increasing regulation and scrutiny are part of everyday social work, as well as limited resources and competing demands, the courage of commitment in practice can be humdrum perhaps more than it is heroic. Again, social workers show integrity when they bring other virtues together, combining care, respectfulness and trustworthiness with justice and courage.

Banks and Gallagher (2009, p. 7) also make the point that the increasing regulation and management of practice means that while virtue ethics has great theoretical appeal, it can be very difficult to apply in practice in the same way that principle-based approaches can be used, as so often seen in codes of ethics. Not only is practice framed by regulations, contracts and standards, but in the contemporary world it is also often experienced as being removed from the ideals of "service". Similarly, Sercombe (2010) argues that there has been a commodification of service, turning a morally informed practice (the professional "serves" the community) into something that can be priced in a market: it becomes "a service".

Yet as the following chapters demonstrate, for those social workers who have developed their character as a social worker through experience, ideas of virtue are a central part of the framework they use to reconsider and articulate the values and ethics of their practice. That these appear differently between individuals is entirely consistent with the contextual understanding of virtues (the qualities of a knife are not those of a clock). For these exemplars of good social work, it becomes clear that virtues in practice cannot be prescriptive. Yet at the same time there is a common language concerning the qualities that are revealed in such accounts of professional life.

For example, in Chap. 2 Sue Ash's narrative reveals courage in dealing with everyday barriers to pursuing valued goals. This is demonstrated in persistence as well as in not only coping with a major life crisis, but using that personal experience subsequently to inform commitments to the service of others that challenged existing structures and practices. In different aspects of her career Sue has also demonstrated the virtue of justice. This is somewhat different to the account in Chap. 8, in that although Bernadette McMenamin's biography presents the same great commitment, persistence and justice, this time it is seen against hostility and overt opposition. Partly this reflects the different areas in which these two social workers have practised. Sue worked in government and non-government child and family services, then subsequently in wider social development roles in the non-government sector. In contrast, Bernadette has spent a career battling the more specific problems of child abuse and sex tourism involving child victims. The more highly controversial field challenges the courage and justice of practitioners in a different way, even though the underlying qualities draw on the same values.

Considering virtue ethics in practice poses a deep question to all members of the profession: what sort of social worker do I wish to be? To return to our metaphor of knives and clocks, some forms of practice may require the quality of sharpness while others necessitate that of steady evenness in progressing through the day. From this it might be expected that different social workers will be able to excel in different areas of the profession, in the sense of their qualities fitting better with the roles involved. The contrast between Sue Ash and Bernadette McMenamin noted above, while drawing on the same ideas of virtue, suggests that such variations are in themselves good as opposed to being a problem for how we might understand virtues in practice.

That they draw on the same range of virtues strengthens this, as it points to the common language of social work concerning the personal qualities of practitioners that is shared across the profession. In this way attention to context and difference is possible without giving ground to a relativism ("anything goes") that undermines the sense of public accountability that professional ethics has to provide. It is in this way that virtue ethics can provide ways of understanding social work values and ethics that, at least according to critics such as McBeath and Webb (2002), is missing from the principle-based ethics that predominate in formal ethical statements (such as codes of ethics). As Banks and Gallagher point out, it is their capacity to be applied in such a way that makes principle-based approaches more "usable" across social structures and systems. Yet without the sense of attention to the context and detail that is offered by virtue ethics, a vital dimension of practice, namely the personal qualities of practitioners, is missing.

Socio-economic and Political Context of Biographies

As indicated above, virtuous action is action that is appropriate to its context. The biographies contained in this book show social workers operating in a wide range of specific situations. But those situations all occurred within a particular temporal and socio-political context, which conditioned both the challenges to which the social workers were responding and the kinds of responses that were available to them. In this section we briefly outline that context.

The social workers whose biographies are contained in this book were born into a society shaped by what has been called the "Australian Settlement". Crafted in the early years of federation at the start of the 20th century, the Australian Settlement involved a kind of compact between organised labour and capital. Its defining features were the "White Australia" policy, "protectionism" of local industry, a centralised industrial relations system and a social welfare system. Protectionism insulated local factory owners from competition by imposing tariffs on imported manufactured goods. The profits consequently achieved by the owners allowed them to pay their workers the "basic wage", which was set by the industrial relations system at a level judged to be sufficient to allow a male worker to support his family in a socially respectable style. The White Australia policy was seen as protection against migration by groups who would be prepared to sell their labour more cheaply than the locals were. Age pensions and unemployment benefits acted as a safety net for those who were unable to find work.

While the Australian Settlement provided the framework for a generally peaceful and cohesive society, in which prosperity was broadly spread, it also institutionalised racial and gender barriers. Labour was divided according to sex, with the presumption that women would marry and devote themselves to running the household and men would go to work to support them, while the White Australia policy reflected accepted views about the hierarchy of races, with the white (Anglo-Saxon) race at the top.

The Australian Settlement reflected the democratic, progressive ethos that emerged in Australia through the 19th and early 20th centuries. That ethos was both promoted and expressed by organised labour, women's organisations and church groups, who agitated for political reform, including women's suffrage, while working to protect the vulnerable and disenfranchised through the provision of free hospitals, women's refuges and schools. Organisations such as the Brotherhood of St Laurence and the Catholic Social Service Bureau, both founded in the 1930s, became (and remain) important providers of social welfare.

Social work as a distinct profession began to emerge in Australia in the late 1920s, informed by the values, knowledge and organisational networks of the activists and workers mentioned in the previous paragraph, as well as by overseas examples. Training courses for "hospital almoners" (in effect, hospital social workers) were established in 1929; social work education subsequently moved into universities, with both Melbourne and Sydney universities setting up social work degrees in 1940.

In 1946 existing state-based organisations co-operated to form the Australian Association of Social Workers (AASW). This organisation has played an important role in advocating for social reform, promoting the interests of its members, and providing a forum for an ongoing and inevitably contentious discussion of the nature of social work. As with the other "caring professions", social work was a highly feminised occupation, both in the gender of the majority of its workforce, and in the way it was regarded—as a kind of hand-maiden to more masculine occupations such as medicine and public administration. Along with similarly placed professions, notably nursing and teaching, the social work profession has struggled to achieve recognition, better pay and conditions, and greater autonomy, over the past decades (Hugman 1991).

The post-war Australia in which members of the AASW plied their trade was a prosperous society, with rising standards of living fuelled by a long economic boom. In the large immigration program established to meet the demand for labour, some 60% of migrants came from non-English speaking countries, moving Australia towards a multicultural society. The welfare state also grew rapidly in this period, with social welfare payments becoming the major item of expenditure of the Commonwealth Government. The demand for social welfare workers, in both government and non-government organisations, saw members of the still-small social work profession—numbering around 500 in the mid-1950s—moving into a range of areas, including child and family welfare, marriage counselling, mental health and probation and prison work. Most of the social workers whose biographies are presented in this book were born and raised during this post-war period, the 1940s and 1950s, and during the peak of their careers they were faced with the end of the post-war consensus and rise of neo-liberalism, discussed further below.

In the last third of the 20th century the elements of the Australian Settlement were dissolved, or at least eroded, in the face of larger social and economic forces, both domestic and international, including the end of the long post-war boom and the rise of neo-liberal ideology among the policy elite. Protectionism began to be wound back in the 1970s, and wage-fixing decentralised in the 1980s. The idea of a "basic wage" to allow for the male breadwinner to provide for his family had become outmoded in a workforce where women were significantly represented, with the two-income family becoming common. With the growth in women's economic power, the norms of marriage and family formation that had held through most of the 20th century weakened. The White Australia policy was overturned in the 1970s, with the quasi-scientific race theory that underpinned it losing all credibility, and a dawning acknowledgement of the reality of Australia's place in Asia. As Australia became more accepting of racial diversity in its migrant intake, it also started to become more sensitive to the need for reconciliation with its Indigenous population.

Over the past 40 years, Australia has changed dramatically, becoming a more dynamic, pluralist and tolerant society. Yet the changes have not been without costs, with a more open economy widening inequality, the "off-shoring" of manufacturing reducing the number of full-time jobs, especially for working-class men, and a buoyant housing market making affordable accommodation elusive for many of the less well-off. While the fundamental problems that social work emerged to address—poverty, social exclusion and dysfunction—remain, the context in which the current social work profession in Australia, now some 30,000 strong (Job Outlook 2012), addresses those problems is more complex than ever. It is important to keep this broad socio-economic and political context in mind while reading the social workers' biographies presented in subsequent chapters.

Method of Choosing Biographies and Analysis

The nature of the research problem, understanding the core virtues of social workers, suggested the suitability of the qualitative research method for the study. Within a narrative research methodology (Liamputtong 2013), a biographical research (Rosenthal 2004) method was employed, as it allowed us to go deep into the professional practice life of social workers and through that process elicit some of the important virtues/qualities (including, roles, life tasks, possible selves, motives, strivings, beliefs, attitudes, values and past experience) that helped them in their practice (see Frey 2010). No other method would have generated such rich data providing deeper insight into practitioners' lives, in the given time frame.

By applying certain criteria such as (1) discernible contribution recognised by the community, (2) some coverage in print and electronic media, (3) minimum ten years of social work practice in the field, (4) representation of gender according to the proportion of female and male social workers, (5) coverage of both urban and rural areas, government and non-government organisations, different practice settings as far as possible, and states and territories according to the spread of AASW membership, a purposive sampling method was employed to select ten social workers whose biographies would be developed (Padgett 2008). Of the ten, eight were females and two were males, three from Victoria, two each from New South Wales and Queensland, and one each from Australian Capital Territory, South Australia and Western Australia.

The method used in the interviews was the Biographic Narrative Interview Method (BNIM) (Wengraf 2001). The core of this research interviewing method is a three sub-session structure. In the first sub-session, a single open-narrative question is asked (all further possible questions are deferred till later) and then the interviewer just supports the interviewee as they improvise an initial overall narrative answer to the question, and then tell the interviewer that they have no more to say. In the second sub-session, the interviewer pushes for more narrative detail on events mentioned, pushes for examples of generalisations made, and in general pushes for Particular Incident Narratives (PINs). In the third (optional) sub-session, all other questions arising from sub-sessions one and two are addressed, narrative or not (see Wengraf 2001, updated in 2016a, b). Clear guidelines and instructions for data collection were developed and provided to all interviewers. As all chief investigators (CIs) were male (though it was not planned in that way), senior female and well-qualified interviewers were recruited to join CIs to conduct co-interviews with respondents. Narrative interviews were digitally recorded, transcribed and examined to ensure the accuracy of the data collected. In addition, secondary data such as resumés, media clippings and online information, where available and relevant to the biographies, were collected. It may be noted that the BNIM's interpretation method was not followed, as it was not needed for the purpose of our study.

The collected narrative biographic data were qualitatively and manually analysed to develop coherent biographies and identify virtues as depicted in narratives. As presented in subsequent chapters, the write-up of each biography included a sequential professional life story followed by discussion of their qualities/character (virtues). Including the four CIs, ten scholars authored these biographies individually and/or jointly.

At a two-day workshop attended by all the authors of biographies and five experts from the fields of philosophy and social work, each biography was presented by its author/s, followed by a focus-group discussion by workshop participants to further analyse each biography and identify virtues, and seek comments and suggestions for improvement. These discussions were digitally recorded and transcribed and qualitatively analysed to identify comments and suggestions, which were communicated to respective authors to further improve biographies and virtue analysis. Further qualitative manual analysis was undertaken to identify common virtues in all ten biographies. The ten biographies presented in this book and the final chapter summarising common virtues are the outcome of this systematic research process.

Some of the limitations of the research approach we employed are the subjective nature of the data collection and analysis process. Although clear criteria were developed to recruit respondents, purposive sampling has recruiters' inbuilt bias. There are many other social workers who would be equally suitable for this study. Identification and analysis of virtues and the choice of events emphasised in the biography may also reflect the researchers' subjectivity and bias. This inevitably meant that from extensive and rich verbatim interviews we had to select the ideas presented in these chapters. Almost all the subjects of biography were senior practitioners and some had retired with an accumulated wealth of practice knowledge. A relatively young practitioner's representation in the research may have been desirable, though such a candidate would have limited experience. With a gender lens, some may point out that all CIs were male in this research, though we balanced it by recruiting female interviewers and co-authors for the biographies. However, such concerns were not raised by any of our respondents. A further limitation of the research is that it does not provide a full description of the organisational contexts within which our subjects worked, and which constrained and informed the decisions they made. We note, however, that our research did typically provide information about the salient features of such contexts, and that in any case (theoretically) the professional autonomy of social workers means that the decisions they make are not determined by the organisational context in which they are made.

Organisation of the Book

This book is organised into 12 chapters. This introductory chapter describes our understanding of the nature of virtue and its role in social work practice, then provides an account of the research methods employed and their limitations, while the final chapter attempts to bring out the synthesis of virtues identified in the ten biographies, the implications of virtue-led practice and its potential application in social work education and training, and practice. Each of the remaining ten chapters contains the biography of a social worker followed by analysis of their virtues. The ten biographies are presented in alphabetical order. The following brief summary may help you choose a biography of interest to you, though of course they may be read in any order. All social workers in these biographies began as ordinary social workers at grassroots level and climbed the ladder of excellence in their own ways, and those ways may lead to further paths for others to follow.

Chapter 2 is a biography of Sue Ash from Western Australia. Sue reflects on 40 years of her professional practice, which shows her leadership in the community services sector, particularly advocacy and policy work, and what social workers are capable of doing.

The biography of Diana Batzias from Victoria is presented in Chap. 3. Diana's 40-year professional career was spread over both government and non-government organisations, introducing significant reforms in both sectors, against many adversities. Diana was described as "quietly unorthodox and a woman of enormous brevity".

Dr. Tom Calma's distinguished professional and public career and his determination to lead, even beyond retirement, and to bring justice to Aboriginal communities stands out in his biography in Chap. 4. Tom is an elder from the Kungarakan and Iwaidja tribal groups from the south-west Darwin region and the Cobourg Peninsula in the Northern Territory. He is based in the Australian Capital Territory.

In Chap. 5 John Gavaghan, a household name in child protection in New South Wales, shows his commitment to clients, unfailing fairness, warmth and good humour, optimism and hope, and an ability to courageously tackle difficult and entrenched issues and to operate reflectively.

Virginia "Ginni" Hall's biography is presented in Chap. 6. From Townsville, Queensland, Ginni is described as a legend by a colleague, and is known for her independence and courage, her dedication and resilience, and her resourcefulness, humanity and humility.

As a rural-based (Orange in New South Wales) grassroots-level practitioner, Bronwyn Hyde's biography in Chap. 7 shows how she emphatically refocused on basics: deep listening, relationship building, locating in the people world and questioning the "taken for granted" assumptions.

Bernadette McMenamin, from Melbourne, Victoria, is the subject of Chap. 8. Her biography describes her social action leading to significant socio-legal change in the field of child sex tourism and abuse. It is insightful to reflect on her resilience and resolve, and her provocative passion.

Chapter 9 is a biography of Dr. Robyn Miller from Victoria. As the Director and Chief Practitioner of the Department of Human Services, Robyn's practice story shows how she supports and inspires professionals to always keep the best interests of children at the centre of decisions.

The story of Dr. Sue Vardon's inspirational career is presented in Chap. 10. Having begun as a social work practitioner, Sue spent 23 years as a chief executive in federal and state governments demonstrated her strength of character and her shrewdness in choice of strategy.

In the final biography, in Chap. 11 Professor Jill Wilson shares her wisdom, explaining how she was driven by concepts of social justice and fairness, a combination of idealism and pragmatism, and a purpose larger than herself.

We present this book of biographies to you with a purpose to inspire you and others to serve better.

References

Alexandra, A., & Miller, S. (2009). *Ethics in practice: Moral theory and the professions*. Sydney: UNSW Press.

Alexandra, A., & Miller, S. (2010). *Integrity systems for occupations*. England: Ashgate.

Annas, J. (2011). *Intelligent virtue*. Oxford: Oxford University Press.

Anscombe, W. (2009). Consilience in social work: Reflections on thinking, doing and being. Ph.D. thesis. Wagga: Charles Sturt University.

Aristotle. (1976). *Nicomachean ethics*. Harmondsworth: Penguin.

Banks, S. (2008). Critical commentary: Social work ethics. *British Journal of Social Work, 38,* 1238–1249.

Banks, S. (2012). *Ethics and values in social work* (3rd ed.). Basingstoke: Palgrave Macmillan.

Banks, S., & Gallagher, A. (2009). *Ethics in professional life: Virtues for health and social care*. Basingstoke: Palgrave Macmillan.

Bowles, W., Collingridge, M., Curry, S., & Valentine, B. (Eds.). (2006). *Ethical practice in social work: An applied approach*. Crows Nest, Sydney: Allen and Unwin.

Clark, C. (2000). *Social work ethics: Politics*. Basingstoke, Macmillan: Principles and Practice.

Clark, C. (2006). Moral character in social work. *British Journal of Social Work, 36,* 75–89.

Coady, N. F., & Wolgien, C. S. (1996). Good therapists' views of how they are helpful. *Clinical Social Work Journal, 24*(3), 311–322.

Cox, D., & Pawar, M. (2013). *International social work: Issues, strategies and programs*. California: Sage.

Edwards, J. A., & Bess, J. M. (1998). Developing effectiveness in the therapeutic use of self. *Clinical Social Work Journal, 26*(1), 89–105.

Egan, G. (2010). *The skilled helper: A problem management and opportunity development approach to helping* (9th ed.). Belmont, CA: Brooks/Cole.

Elliott, C. (2000). Tuning and practicing the therapeutic instrument: The therapist's life experience. *Clinical Social Work Journal, 28*(3), 321–330.

Frey, W. (2010). Teaching virtue: Pedagogical implications of moral psychology. *Science and Engineering Ethics, 16,* 611–628.

Furrow, D. (2005). *Ethics: Key concepts in philosophy*. New York: Continuum.

Gray, M. (2010). Moral sources and emergent ethical theories in social work. *British Journal of Social Work, 40,* 1794–1811.

Gray, M., & Webb, S. A. (2009). *Social work theories and methods*. London: Sage.

Healy, K. (2005). *Social work theories in context: Creating frameworks in practice*. Basingstoke: Palgrave/Macmillan.

Healy, K. (2012). *Social work methods and skills*. Basingstoke: Palgrave Macmillan.

Hepworth, D. H., Rooney, R. H., & Larsen, J. A. (2002). *Direct social work practice*. Pacific Grove: Brooks/Cole.

Hornby, A. S. (1992). *Oxford advanced learners dictionary*. Oxford: Oxford University Press.

Houston, S. (2003). Establishing virtue in social work: A response to McBeath and Webb. *British Journal of Social Work, 33,* 819–824.

Howe, D. (2009). *A brief introduction to social work theory*. Basingstoke: Palgrave/Macmillan.

Hugman, R. (1991). *Power in caring professions*. London: Macmillan.

Hugman, R. (2005). *New approaches in ethics for caring professions*. Basingstoke: Palgrave/Macmillan.

Hugman, R., & Smith, D. (1995). Ethical issues in social work: An overview. In R. Hugman & D. Smith (Eds.), *Ethical issues in social work* (pp. 1–15). London: Routledge.

Job Outlook. (2012). Social workers. http://joboutlook.gov.au/occupation.aspx?search=alpha&tab=prospects&code=2725. Accessed 26 October 2016.

Kant, I. (1964). *The groundwork of the metaphysics of morals*. New York: Harper & Row.

Liamputtong, P. (2013). *Qualitative research methods* (4th ed.). Melbourne: Oxford University Press.

MacIntyre, A. (1998). *A short history of ethics*. Notre Dame: University of Notre Dame Press.

McBeath, G., & Webb, S. A. (2002). Virtue ethics and social work: Being lucky, realistic, and not doing one's duty. *British Journal of Social Work, 32,* 1015–1036.

Miller, C. (2014). The problem of character. In S. van Hooft (Ed.), *The handbook of virtue ethics*. New York: Routledge.

Mowbray, M. (1996). Community work practice and a case for the renovation of community work education. *Australian Social Work, 49*(2), 3.

Padgett, D. K. (2008). *Qualitative methods in social work research*. Thousand Oaks: Sage.

Pawar, M., & Anscombe, A. W. (2015). *Reflective social work practice: Thinking, doing and being*. Melbourne: Cambridge University Press.

Payne, M. (2005). *Modern social work theory*. Basingstoke: Palgrave/Macmillan.

Pullen-Sansfacon, A. (2010). Virtue ethics for social work: A new pedagogy for practical reasoning. *Social Work Education, 29*(4), 402–415.

Reupert, A. (2006). The counsellor's self in therapy: An inevitable presence. *The International Journal for the Advancement of Counselling, 28*(1), 95–105.

Rosenthal, G. (2004). Biographical research. In C. Seale, G. Gobo, J. F. Gubrium, & D. Silverman (Eds.), *Qualitative research practice*. London: Sage.

Sercombe, H. (2010). *Youth work ethics*. London: Sage Publications.

Teater, B. (2010). *An introduction to applying social work theories and methods*. New York: Oxford University Press.

Webb, S. (2010). Virtue ethics. In M. Gray & S. A. Webb (Eds.), *Ethics and value perspectives in social work* (pp. 108–119). Basingstoke, England: Palgrave Macmillan.

Wengraf, T. (2001). *Qualitative research interviewing: Biographic narrative and semi-structured methods*. London: Sage.

Wengraf, T. (2016a). *BNIM quick outline sketch.* (Author's updated notes available from tom.wengraf@gmail.com).

Wengraf, T. (2016b). *BNIM short guide and detailed manual.* (Author's updated notes available from tom.wengraf@gmail.com).

Chapter 2
Voice to the Voiceless—Sue Ash, AO

Christina Fernandes and Richard Hugman

"Sue Ash speaks up for the voiceless", "Coming out as gay in the country" and "Community at a crossroads": these media articles highlight the advocacy and policy work of Sue Ash, AO, a well-known Western Australian leader in the community services sector. After more than 40 years of experience in this sector, Sue reflects on the context in which contemporary social work is situated, a *different environment ... with statutory compliance like we've never had before ... with legal sanctions like we've never had before ... with an increasing disrespect for our human services and ... we're becoming agents of some very draconian policy.* She ponders on the future of social work and *how we actually keep a profession alive when most of our salaries are coming from the public sector*, grateful of her membership of the non-profit sector where *we can value social work.*

The interview came at a turning point in Sue's life—the recent loss of her mother and increasing caring responsibilities for her father. A time to once again look and plan for the future, acknowledging how the past has shaped her and that she is now at a time where she is content with her *professional voice* and her contribution to the profession: *over the last few years it's been great to own being a social worker and try and put something back into both our profession but also for the world actually seeing what social workers are capable of doing.*

C. Fernandes (✉)
Curtin University, Perth, Australia
e-mail: C.Fernandes@curtin.edu.au

R. Hugman
University of New South Wales, Sydney, Australia
e-mail: r.hugman@unsw.edu.au

M. Pawar et al. (eds.), *Empowering Social Workers*,
DOI 10.1007/978-981-10-3809-9_2

Early Life

This was a family where you could talk about things.

A deep sense of community and civic-mindedness, instilled and embodied by Sue's parents, are enduring influences in her life. These virtues were necessary in the *isolated little community* that was Middle Swan, Western Australia, in 1951. The family in which Sue grew up was one where membership and involvement in the Christian church and the sense of responsibility to contribute to the wellbeing of the community lay at the core. It is clear that these family values were, and still are, a significant influence in Sue's personal and professional life.

Although the eldest of three, Sue was an *innately shy* child: so much so that Jill, her younger sister by two and a half years, was *the voice for the pair* of them on shopping errands and in other public activities. *We would go to the shops together, as you did in those days, at four and a half and two, and it would be Jill who would order the sausages.* The family knew this but, importantly, Sue was never made to feel different or incapable for this almost excruciating shyness—she was accepted and loved just as she was. She was not subjected to the labelling or categorisation that she feels defines contemporary childhood, but rather left to grow at her own pace. And a capable and confident Sue took on the role of carer, with responsibilities in the home, and for her mum during her *really nasty pregnancies*. Being *very competent at home but not competent outside* meant that Sue's career success has been somewhat of a surprise to her.

Sue's mother, Joan—what we would now call a "stay-at-home mum" but what was the norm at the time—played a pivotal role in Sue's life. Her sacrifice of career and independence for family life was common for women of that generation. Her enforced relinquishment of a job as a public servant and subsequent need to rear a family on the outskirts of Perth meant she needed to find something else to keep her sane: finding a niche in the community and Methodist church provided this and also instilled in her children an understanding of the importance of participating in civic life. Looking after the children on her own while her husband was away for work, *catching the bus once a week to see her mother* and being involved in the church kept Joan busy and connected in a small community.

A man of his times, Sue's father, Ross, held more black and white attitudes than Joan, but he too held a strong belief in community and Christian faith. A self-employed builder by trade and necessity, Ross held aspirations for a career in civil engineering that proved elusive, for the course he had worked hard and nearly completed was not accredited. Sue recalls this as being soul destroying for her father, for all the years of studying at night and travelling for work had in the end not achieved the university degree that he'd aimed for. Instead he continued as a builder, the family moving multiple times for him to secure employment.

Significantly, these were parents who enacted their civic-mindedness. Within months of being married they were sharing their house and spare room with Dutch refugees who couldn't find accommodation. Caring for and about others was *part of our narrative in our family and [the family was] always expected to do things like that.* The family always had a world perspective and an involvement in overseas missionary activities. A formative part of childhood that Sue loved was staying up late, listening to the cricket in England (on a crystal set), and imagining a world across the seas. This contact with the outside world came to a head when, as a ten-year-old, Sue listened aghast to stories of the brutal fight for independence in Belgian Congo. This was a turning point for her, as she learned firstly about the human potential for good and bad, *for good people to do some pretty awful things.* It was also the beginnings of the development of a complex and nuanced understanding of white privilege. Although *this was a family where you could talk about things* Sue felt confused and confronted and held her thoughts privately, unable and unprepared to talk to anyone about them, but knowing somehow that her life in sleepy Western Australia had changed forever.

The Sue at school was the Sue in public: a quiet achiever in primary school, but who spent many hours in the high school library until a librarian coaxed her out at lunchtimes; this teacher, like other influential people in Sue's life, went on to become and remain a friend over many years. The 1960s were a time when girls studied domestic science and boys technical drawing; Sue wanted to be an architect and the pathway for that was technical drawing, one that was closed to her simply due to her gender. Demure, quiet Sue performed her first act of civil disobedience at being *told that as a girl I couldn't do it. I had to do domestic science.* With a satisfied smile on her face, Sue recounts sitting in the playground letting the sponge cake burn: *I know I can make a sponge but there's no way in the world I'm going to allow you to have the last laugh.*

And so school lost some meaning for Sue until year 11, for being unable to learn technical drawing and related subjects had a significant effect on her, her results becoming *pretty ordinary.* Yet another change in schools, this time to enable her to go on to year 12, which her family supported, despite their meagre resources. Making the most of teenage life meant that Sue's marks suffered and, so strong was her sense of responsibility in not letting her parents or herself down, she decided that she would leave school and train in dental nursing. Although her family *knew that I wasn't going to last,* having felt so much compassion for her sister Jill that she fainted regularly on seeing Jill in pain in the dentist's chair, they allowed her to make the choice. Lasting only six weeks in this respectable and suitable job for a woman, Sue *plucked up the courage* to tell her parents she wanted to return to school. Although the financial costs incurred in buying uniform and equipment for dental nursing were significant, her parents supported this decision. She returned to school to year 12 and it was at this point that Sue encountered economics and her love for the subject.

Starting Out in Social Work

> The early 1960s for me were really big years because they were years where I was … yeah, I was just doing a whole pile of thinking … and appreciated the opportunity of being able to belong to Perth …

Without any sense of what she wanted to do, at the suggestion of a school counsellor in 1968, at the age of 16, Sue applied for, and successfully obtained, two cadetships, one with the Department of Child Welfare and one into engineering with Main Roads. She chose social work because in order to do engineering she would have had to do extra work to make up for not studying physics at school, and she and her family were travelling during that period. Sue also refers to herself at this time as being *somewhat of a feminis*t; it's no wonder then that social work was *a joy*, opening up *a whole new world.* Social work at the Western Australian Institute of Technology (WAIT), now Curtin University, was thus a breath of fresh air, a formative period of learning about social economics, anthropology and community. It was also a time when Sue questioned what she saw as a mismatch between the social justice she read of in the Bible and its absence in her church. As an adolescent she *couldn't join the two together* and *social work for me was a really wonderful opportunity to have a different world view on justice ... it also equipped me to see the world through a whole range of different people's ... world views would be the language we use these days.*

The social work course was an opportunity for Sue to learn about politics *in a systemic way*, to *see the world through community as well as individuals.* It was also an opportunity to find her own voice in a period when she was treated as though she was capable, despite her age. Sue speaks of the different, lower status accorded to WAIT courses because at that time it had just moved from a technical to a degree course, saying she was *really delighted to be at WAIT because there's nothing that fires me up like being told that you're not good enough.* It was this voice that enabled Sue's resistance tot being told that WAIT social work students could not do medical social work placements. At the encouragement of a WAIT social work lecturer, Sue and a colleague travelled to New Zealand to complete their final placements, not only a medical placement but a four-month psychiatric medical social work placement. Speaking of this period, Sue says, *It was quite important to both of us to actually find a way through the system to actually achieve what we wanted to do.* This was also the beginning of a lifetime of travel; social work has been a *wonderful career for a woman who wanted to travel ... rather than just being a tourist.*

The other opportunity for Sue to test her voice was when she and other students felt that the therapeutic processes in which they were compelled to participate were traumatic to some. This was *the era of therapeutic communities and we had all these amazing in-depth focus groups where you would bare all and sometimes you would feel as though you were being torn apart and not put back together very well.* At 19 Sue was nearing the point of withdrawing from the course—a big decision, given her love and commitment to social work knowledge. She shared these thoughts with her mother, who *rarely intervened in our lives* and, spurred on by her mother's uncharacteristic threat of going into talk to the Head of Department, Sue took matters into her own hands. She challenged the lecturer *about his boundaries* and the *pulling [the person] apart* which felt *almost gratuitous.* It was this experience that taught her the importance of fully informed consent, a value she has held dear through her career: *What should have happened, and what I always endeavoured to do from then on, is to ensure that we demonstrate full consent.*

The feminist movement was influential in Sue *finding her voice*, standing up against the school system that prevented her from pursuing technical drawing, the hierarchy between the two social work courses, and the lecturer who she felt *abused his power with vulnerable women.* Of this period Sue describes herself as not being so much a *public feminist of the seventies* and *your ordinary feminist* but that *the essence of being feminist was absolutely there.* Although different today, being a feminist in the church was *interesting*: but then Sue *always intended to push boundaries.*

Social Work Placements

> Over the years what were opportunities to learn new things gradually became integrated and it's been a really strong part of my personal development to live an integrated life…

Sue's placement opportunities were diverse: City of South Perth (community survey); Mofflyn, now UnitingCare West; and Catholic Migration, now Centrecare.

It was this last placement with Barry Hickey—who later became Archbishop of Perth—that Sue, a 19-year-old, worked with a poor Irish working family on managing their budget. One Friday, six weeks later, she called into their house to find (non-budgeted) fish and chips on the kitchen table. It was here that Sue learned something more about poverty and that *we're much more than rational beings.* She speaks of the importance of learning from clients, who are the experts in their own lives. While her immediate reaction was to wonder why and how the family made the decision to splurge when they *were doing so well*, later, when she was driving home, she had the realisation that:

> these people wanted to ensure that their children had a normal experience and they … you know, the short-term consequences versus the long-term pain, they'd lived in poverty a long time. They probably knew a million more times than their 19-year-old social worker about how they would do that. But it was so important for them that their kids had something special and for them special was fish and chips.

Sue says: *the history of my career is you just (keep) learning … it was just a powerful lesson.*

Sue completed her final exams on her twentieth birthday; that is, she was considered young; when the subject of the appropriate age to study social work arises on social work advisory groups she challenges this, saying *I had a demonstrated capacity to learn and I think some of the really critical things that have formed me as a social worker were already well formed by the time I was twenty.*

Early Career

> Work has never really been a hardship because it's always been ... I don't know that it's quite vocation but it's certainly been a career or a profession rather than a job.

The finance section of the Department of Child Welfare was to be Sue's first job, where at 17 her role was to process foster care payments, *which for someone with a brain like mine took a lot of discipline because I was much more interested in figuring out where the money went than making sure all the numbers added up.* Once again she speaks of the influence of a mentor, Mike, who later became a friend: a *fantastic public servant* who built into her a *sense of responsibility* that if you get it wrong you will impact someone's life. It was Mike who taught her about what public service means and the art of translation that she believes is essential for social work: *he took what I learnt about politics and he translated it for me.* Sue reflects on how they worked with paper, where clients had cards that were *tangible evidence* and helped social workers understand *how critical their work was in those days because they weren't an entry on the screen.* She learned an important lesson: *get it right and you're part of a really well-oiled machine that's providing good care for a child.*

Family welfare officers, though considered a lower rank than social workers, also mentored and guided Sue, showing her how to do everyday administrative tasks as well as about accountability in a legal environment. Speaking of their openness and warm welcome, she cites her thirst for learning: *I'm sure my curiosity helped because I wasn't there under sufferance. I really wanted to know.* One officer, also a good friend now, coached and modelled for her how to stick to a decision once you had made it, that her job was to protect the life of vulnerable children. This helped her in an early recommendation as a worker in adoptions, rejecting a prospective adoptive family's care application and being able to articulate the reasons for her verdict. It was also at this time that Sue learned two valuable lessons: *track the money* and that *process has always only ever been about ensuring that you get good outcomes, respectful outcomes for your employer but good outcomes for people and those sort of process things are not the end point.* It was these mentors in her life who enabled her to see that effective social workers *understand where the money is, who makes the decisions and how it transfers.* Effective social workers are aware of their power and the mindful and judicious use of this power: *Don't assume anybody wants you in their life. They need you in their life because of your position. So don't abuse it. Don't do any harm and if you feel as though you're doing harm, stand back.*

Social work enabled travel and Sue made the most of these opportunities, travelling to Kalgoorlie and Esperance in her role as adoptions officer, staying with work colleagues who became friends, friends she still has today. An experience in this role had a resounding effect, *I still can't drive down this street in Perth without remembering this child.* Well into the adoption process, the birth mother revoked her consent and 20-year-old Sue *had to go and get this baby* from the adoptive parents. The support she received helped her, for she *learnt about the consequences of decisions without feeling as though I was being clobbered because we made a wrong decision.* She was involved again later when the same child came into care and she has been a colleague to the mother of the second adoptive family, highlighting once again the importance of integration of personal and professional aspects of self: *We've had this intertwining (personal/professional) relationship and for me the only way you get through that is this integration of your self.*

At age 22 Sue spent two years at the new combined department called Community Welfare in Derby, in far north Western Australia, working with colleagues to develop Aboriginal communities and in collaboration with all the state government agencies. She notes that her learning there was *how fantastic it is to actually work across a team and not just a team in an organisation, but across the community.* Sue was involved in the early stages of the development of the community at One Arm Point, with the Bardi people; she worked with the elders in the Indigenous communities who *were incredibly gracious of this little white girl.* It was here that Sue had another life-changing experience, this time with an Indigenous child who she brought to Perth from Derby for adoption. Of her role in this Sue says, *I wasn't part of all the decision making but I was a critical part of her [relinquishing Aboriginal parent] losing her son.* For Sue, *the line between child protection and Stolen Generation, even as late as the early seventies, was still very blurred.* Years later, at a Bringing Them Home conference, she worked with an Indigenous leader on a shared presentation as a way to work through social work's involvement with the Stolen Generation. Of this time Sue says, *And I really wanted to represent colleagues, me included, in what I think was a very ambivalent period in social work practice. And to be absolutely honest I think we are still there but we coat it with all sorts of other things.* Sue's hope is to one day return to the Kimberly to meet the mother: *I think I'm brave enough now that if she's really angry about what happened and that she didn't get her son back or something awful happened that I can probably cope with that.*

Sue also speaks of the two-storey office building in Derby, which *literally looked down on the reserve … I was always uncomfortable ... because it just spoke privilege.* Yet this bird's eye view also meant that staff could see what was happening in the community and meant that *you didn't need to intrude on people's lives.* Sue sums this up when she says: *I think that whole sense of trying not to abuse privilege but being curious is a really interesting challenge for us as people who work with people.*

Sound observational skills, many of which seem to be lost today, were developed early in Sue's training and practised in Derby in a multicultural situation:

> In the era that I was trained in, all of us were great people observers. We would go to dinner and we would make up the story of the person at the next table and you would practise your nonverbal observation and you'd practise your interpretation of dress and code and all those sorts of things. We just did it all the time.

Not only was working in the Kimberley an amazing opportunity to fly over and visit beautiful parts of Western Australia, it was a chance to practise preventative work, keeping families together, and without paternalistic state responses. An example of this was a girl who was placed in foster care during the week while her single-parent father was at work. Comparing it to more rigid contemporary responses Sue says:

> We'd probably call it shared care these days but for the Dad, he saw himself as still being her primary carer but he was just supported by another couple and for his daughter, she literally moved from his place to their place and back again and it was all very normal. I grieve the fact that we find it so difficult to do those things these days … today … she would have been in care.

Unhappy with being rejected for a senior position for which she concedes she was not professionally ready, Sue decided not to return to Derby after a trip to Perth for medical treatment. She decided that after a visit to Papua New Guinea to see her parents she would continue to England. However, this trip did not eventuate; the lure of another rural job based with an aerial health service, establishing health centres in outback New South Wales, proved too strong. Newcastle was to become Sue's next home base and a multidisciplinary work team environment was one in which she flourished. The team travelled to Broken Hill and Lightning Ridge and Brewarrina and Albury and anywhere that was outback New South Wales. When the team was moved to Sydney, Sue chose to find another job in Newcastle, from where she could visit Sydney but avoid the hassle of living in a big city.

This was the Whitlam era, and the next phase of Sue's life, at the NSW Department of Social Services, involved regional community development work. Now part of the Newcastle community, she and a friend became aware of the increasing rates of domestic violence as a result of the downsizing of the BHP iron works. They travelled to Sydney to see Elsie Women's Refuge and to Canberra to see the newly established refuge there, returning to form Jenny House, a *little project on the side* of their day jobs that in reality involved intricate and lengthy consultation, collaboration and negotiation with business and local government.

Sue transferred back to Perth to the Midland Department of Social Security. Although the idea was to spend a year with her sister and brother (who were both getting married at the end of the year) and then travel to England, the plan was thwarted, but for good reason: it was at Midland that Sue met Graeme, who she subsequently married and with whom she had two children. To support Graeme's subsequent studies in agriculture prior to training for the Uniting Church ministry, Sue worked as a consultant for five years. They were not able to fulfil their hope to work in rural/remote Australia, for Graeme died suddenly in 1986, at the age of 29, only nine years into their marriage.

Now a single parent and primary breadwinner with two children under the age of six, Sue experienced being a "client", becoming acutely aware of the *little symbols of power* manifested, for example, in the quality of waiting rooms and reception areas and separate staff and client entrances. Sue had always been aware of the importance of knowing how fine the line was between "provider" and "consumer", that *today you could be in one seat and tomorrow you could be in another*. These new experiences reinforced her belief that *If you have been given the privilege of a position then function as though it's a privilege and not a right, and function as though the person you're working with could easily be in the same circumstance that you are and you could be in their circumstance.* These experiences informed her current view that *clients are treated as well or better than staff,* which means that *client areas need to be as good as your staff areas.* Staff need equal focus for *our staff do amazingly difficult jobs and they need to know that they're valued and looked after and cared for.*

Another aspect of the personal and professional influencing each other was the awareness for Sue of the importance of children's involvement in *the reality* of death and how her grief, although deep, was different to that of many social work clients, for whom grief was multiple. Sue reflects on her positioning of herself as *fortunate,* saying:

> I was a well-educated 34-year-old with two kids. I mean, you cannot get a bigger sympathy vote than me. But, you know there would be people who wouldn't get the support that I got or people who would deal with it differently or people who hadn't had my social work background and I cannot tell you how important that was.

Graeme's death meant that Sue had to make some life-changing decisions in her professional life; after trying to manage part-time work with vulnerable families she decided that these families needed a social worker who was able to provide support and skills and she was not yet ready to provide that. And so began the first of a series of ten-year life plans to sort decisions about life and work.

A Graduate Diploma in Primary Teaching, though on the plan, was not for Sue and seven weeks later she applied for and successfully obtained a full-time lecturing position at TAFE, teaching in her area of expertise—out-of-home care for kids and working with children with disabilities. This position enabled her to combine parenting and employment and was something Sue had always wanted to do. It was during this time that she feels she had one of her greatest achievements: seeing 22 out of 23 Indigenous students graduate from an inclusion course that she had worked on at its inception. Sue puts it down to the students: *these students were generous with their sharing of knowledge and culture and I think we really built a community in that group.*

By this time Sue had also taken on a leadership role in her church and obtained a Diploma in Theology. Her faith, though tested, has guided her through the majority of her adult life. Her first period of questioning Christianity was during universit, when she queried where the espoused social justice was manifested in the church. Years later, in Newcastle in the Department of Social Services, as the only Protestant on the team, Sue was exposed to different ways of thinking. Derby had already been in a point in her life when she had decided that the Christian faith, although appropriate for her parents, was not for her. Her parents' response that they accepted her decision and would be praying for her angered her *because I think deep in my own personal belief system there was an acknowledgement of the power of God and if they were praying then no matter what they did behaviourally there was still influence.* It was during some time off a few years later, ironically while working in a pest control agency, that Sue reflected on the importance of Christian faith and, after much consideration, *came to grips with a personal Christian faith and that has been really solid since then.*

Education continued to play a key role when Sue was involved in setting up a regional social work course at Edith Cowan University in Bunbury, Western Australia, bringing together two passions: social work and regional communities. She returned to an operational position as a manager in the Department of Family and Community Services, once again covering regional WA. The position required extensive travel and the family perfected *Telstra parenting*—doing many family activities via phone calls. This was the first of a series of senior management jobs in Sue's career. She was able to once again *join the dots*: her boss from Derby was her boss at FaCS in Bunbury. Departure from that position due to a restructure was postponed by a significant local disaster: a landslide in 1996 in the coastal town of Gracetown involved managing a multi-community recovery effort, working in a team of police, fire fighters and health professionals. Another learning opportunity: Sue regrets her assumption that she knew what the families needed; she provided privacy in their time of grief when what they needed, they later said, was community.

> I was applying this sense of being an individual in grief and shock and wanting … not applying learning around self-determination but doing what you think is right for the person as opposed to enabling people to engage in decision making, even in what was a really difficult set of circumstances for these people.

Gracetown also had a *big impact ... in terms of always working with rather than doing to and enabling people to have as much opportunity to make decisions for themselves as they possibly can and that communities are different to aggregates of individuals.* It was at this point that Sue learned the importance of being bilingual and knowing and understanding concepts well enough to translate them into other people's professional language. After all, it is a social worker's *systemic ecological understanding of the world* to be respectful of languages and cultures.

Leadership

Sue's qualities as a leader were further strengthened in her first position as Chief Executive Officer, at Wanslea (Family Services). For a period of seven years she oversaw the threefold growth of the organisation and the establishment of regional facilities. Mission and value changes were developed as well, and a broader definition of family, current to the twentieth century, was applied to the constitution. A move from a traditional conceptualisation of family as confined to mother and child to one that was *broader ... multiple generations, multiple gender, all sorts of things.* This enabled opportunities for the creation of *programs for grandparents caring for grandchildren, for family members who were no longer with custody of their kids, with fathers, with children caring for parents.* Computerisation of client records and the creation of a client data system enabled a research focus that was absent in other agencies at this time. It was also a time of personal growth for Sue, who never saw herself as a leader, equating quietness with an inability to be a leader. Learning around leadership was significant, with the realisation that *if you can build a team and you can build a vision and a direction and you can ask the right questions you can actually shape things.*

With her children grown up, it was time for a change, this time to Canberra to be Manager of Child Protection for the ACT Government. A review of the child protection system commenced soon after and a significant period of flux ensued over the next year. Returning to Perth to be closer to an ill father and to return to education, Sue commenced work as a lecturer at Curtin University, where she had started her education more than 35 years before. The pressures of extensive teaching, a PhD, less income and a sense that the contribution she was making was minimal, led her to resign from Curtin to take a position as CEO of an aged care organisation for which she had been head-hunted. Three years later, Sue moved to the position of CEO, WA Council of Social Service (WACOSS).

WACOSS was to become Sue's *Esther job*, a two–and-half-year job that enabled all the elements in her life to integrate. Dealing with the media was a steep learning curve and she established a strategy that addressed both the general citizen (people like her own mother) and senior government decision makers. Once again Sue grew an agency, expanding it within the context of an extremely tight budget.

Participating in the local and Australian community through volunteer work has always been part of Sue's life: the establishment of Families Australia, involvement with the Australian Family Support Association and membership, including presidency, of WACOSS and membership of the Board of ACOSS. Giving back to those who had supported her and her family was equally important, as was contributing to the Uniting Church ministry with whom Graeme had been training when he died and whose insurance policy had enabled Sue to put a deposit on her first home. Sue speaks of her philosophy around volunteer work as being *typical of my career... There's always been voluntary projects on the backend of various things that I've done because again I think you're given much and it's a great opportunity to see what you can do with it.*

In April 2010, Sue proposed to the WACOSS Board that WACOSS become the local partner with the Commonwealth Foundation on the delivery of the Commonwealth People's Forum (CPF) during the Commonwealth Heads of Government Meetings (CHOGM) in October 2011. This involved 18 months of work, including significant international leadership and negotiation. Delivery of the CPF was a highlight of Sue's career. This was an opportunity to influence what was to go on in the national social policy debate of CHOGM and to demonstrate to the state government what WACOSS could contribute. Two thousand Western Australian citizens were directly involved in some aspect of the CPF. Of this *little bit busy* period Sue says, *I suppose for me just that growing personal sense of confidence about being able to lead and influence and build teams and work with some amazing people*. A significant, though quiet achievement, was facilitating the presentation by three Indigenous elders to Kevin Rudd, then Prime Minister, Australian foreign minister, and all the foreign ministers. For this and her other work Sue received an Officer of the Order of Australia (AO) in 2014, for "distinguished service to the community, particularly in the area of social policy development, reform and implementation, and to the provision of services to people in need". This was a major achievement for a quiet girl from Middle Swan, yet Sue shows her humility by saying that her happiness is from the joy that it gave other people in the sector and that it was the first time many people actually knew someone on the list. This award came as *both a surprise and a huge honour and again, for me, the personal and the professional collided.* During the lead-up to CHOGM Sue moved to her current position of CEO of UnitingCare West, which was another agency that nurtured the integration of all the spheres of her life. Sue took this job because of the social justice part of the agency, its faith base and its intentionality about its mission.

The Future for Social Work

> We're a profession of hope and opportunity and justice … so let's use all that we've got and set some long horizons and then work towards them.

For Sue, the future for social work is one in which we recognise our *responsibility to challenge systems* and alongside our strengths of description and critiquing, we also have to develop an ability to find and provide *alternative solutions*, many of which involve the *awful inevitable problem of compromising.*

No matter what Sue does for the next ten years, it is clear she will continue to be a leader, because her style of leadership is one needed for social workers struggling in the current context. Leadership is about being able to develop and nurture people's abilities, *about building capability and treating people as capable.* It is about being aware of not letting your ego get too big, of being open: *interested and ... curious and understanding there may be additional aspects to issues that you really need to be taking into account as you form your opinion.*

Analysis of Qualities/Character

Integrity: Joining the Dots

In considering the expression of values and character in her life narrative, Sue Ash presents an overarching theme of the integration of the personal and the professional self. This is seen clearly in her account of *joining the dots.* At one point this is explained in terms of *joining the applied with the theory, joining the policy with the practice, joining the international with the national and joining the individual with the community* (points to which the discussion returns below). These ideas convey a sense of integration of thinking and action that is constantly attending to the complexities and contradictions of the world. In contrast, for Sue *joining the dots* also means personal integrity. She says *I started to see my career [in terms of the] joining bits of my passions*. Again, this notion appears in a practical sense in a commitment to making different parts of a role fit together. But most of all it means being able to hold the different aspects of oneself in a coherent whole, so that beliefs and values are expressed coherently in practices and relationships. Examples of what this looked like in day-to-day practice include the use of *plain language*, so that people of different cultural and educational backgrounds could understand what was happening. As Sue puts it:

> I would privilege plain language and the capacity to engage people with me in the thinking rather than use exclusionary language which would give me more power in some environments but not in others. I thought how can you have all this knowledge and understanding and espouse self-determination and inclusion and then function exactly the opposite to that? It never resonated … it didn't sit well with me.

A personal quality that Sue brings to her professional role is her Christian faith and she considers that her current role as CEO of UnitingCare West permits this to feel more directly integrated, yet the values she espouses and demonstrates are congruent with this belief system. Indeed, in one account from her early life she describes how she became aware that Christian theology often makes strong pronouncements about social justice while at the same time church institutions fail to act on this value. As she says, *I couldn't see it being enacted in the churches I was part of*. While at that stage she sought to achieve greater integrity by moving away from religious belief, over time as faith increasingly became an important foundation for her own life, her response was to put effort into trying to change church institutions from the inside. This has involved voluntary work throughout her life. It also forms the backdrop to the integration of all aspects of Sue's identity and her relationships—in social work, in her family and in the community (including the church). Together, these qualities identify the integration of the personal and the professional as a way of developing and maintaining congruence in values and purpose, which characterises the whole of Sue's account of her career and life.

Thus, to the observer, Sue's character can be summarised in the expression "what you see is what you get". Sometimes such a description can be used to portray a person who is inflexible and perhaps unreflective, whereas Sue is the opposite of this. What she displays is openness and consideration of others, combined with consistency, reliability and intentionality. Sue reports how in her early adult life she was described by a supervisor as "stolid" and that she baulked at this, feeling it was *not an easy word to hear*. Yet she puts this into context by saying that she would have preferred to be described as *reasonable and responsible and competent and capable*, all of which might point to a personal strength and maturity, which it is possible this supervisor was trying to communicate.

Within the interviews there are some values that are particularly strongly expressed and form the substance of what it might be said Sue integrates from a moral or ethical perspective. These are: social justice, power and responsibility, commitment and resilience, and a broader set of values that together contribute complexity and detail to the whole picture. So these will now be discussed in more detail.

Social Justice

The expression of social justice as a core value runs throughout Sue's life narrative. Her memory of her family providing accommodation for a refugee family in the early 1950s is combined with a childhood awareness of being white and the privilege that this conferred in a society such as Australia. Ironically, this latter understanding came from listening to world news of the implications of decolonisation in Africa and the atrocities being experienced by colonists in the Congo. It was not that Sue had a sense of entitlement through whiteness, but rather the empirical observation that it came with privilege and a realisation that in other circumstances to those of her own life this was being challenged. This then helped her to develop a deeper understanding of what "racial" constructions of life opportunities might involve.

Alongside this developing understanding was also a realisation that human beings, *[even] good people [could] do some pretty awful things [when put] in circumstances of survival or whatever*. This has been a life-long lesson, as *to this day it still impacts me what people can do to each other* but, moreover, *this wasn't just about the other [as] I was probably in some circumstances capable of doing the same thing*.

As noted above, Sue had also learned as a teenager that the ideas people express and their actions may not always be congruent, as she had been impressed with the biblical theme of social justice, while in the relationships and structures of the churches that she had attended she had not observed the value being acted on. At this stage she rejected faith as the basis for such values and held on to the idea of social justice. This she found supported by social work studies, especially in subjects such as anthropology, economics and politics. She also encountered aspects of injustice in her own situation, both as a woman and as someone who was studying at a non-university institution. For example, particular parts of social work were closed off as options for practice placements (field education). These became factors that Sue found ways of challenging, and thus they became important lessons in struggling with injustice, whether on grounds of gender or of social class. This resonated with her earlier experience of being blocked from doing technical drawing at school because as a girl she had to do domestic science—she had practised a form of resistance by deliberately not doing well (letting a cake burn). Later in her life the same commitment has been expressed in participating in the establishment of a women's refuge in Newcastle and in being part of the Women's Electoral Lobby.

For example, as CEO of WACOSS a particular achievement was in working with the Premier of Western Australia to ensure that when the CHOGM took place in Perth four significant social justice goals were included in the agenda. First, that there was Indigenous leadership represented at the meeting; second, to ensure that homeless people in the city were not harmed by the various logistical and security arrangements that were put in place; third, that refugees' and migrants' issues were placed on the agenda; and fourth, that mental health and trauma were also considered. In doing this, the political dimension of social justice was brought to the forefront as part of the social work role. Thus the role of WACOSS CEO enabled Sue to act on what for her is both a personal and a professional core value.

Power and Responsibility

As Sue has progressed through her career her sense of social justice has become much more concrete and immediate. The first example that she describes is the experience of being a social worker in the Kimberley, and her encounter with service users from a different cultural background. She became aware that power took the form of language as well as of the capacity to make decisions affecting other people's lives. In this sense language meant both a particular usage of English and also the use of technical, professional concepts. This is the power of control through exclusion. She realised this was the antithesis of the core social work principles of inclusion and self-determination.

A major point in this respect was from her experiences when her husband died and she found herself as a service user at this very vulnerable point. *I went from being a senior social worker in the Department of Social Services to a client and I remember sitting in the waiting room ... and the sense of the little symbols of power were very strong.* Subsequently this understanding that the relationship between professionals and service users is basically one of power has affected all aspects of her work. This can be seen in three particular ways that Sue regards good practice: power exercised in one's own practice; the responsibilities that professionals have towards service users arising from the power that is exercised; and, more broadly, that professionalism is about service.

In respect to the exercise of power in her own work, Sue expresses this in very tangible ways. For example, in her early work in child welfare she learned that quite mundane aspects of interaction with service users, such as processing payments accurately and on time, could impact dramatically on the lives of disadvantaged people. So what some professionals might regard as bureaucracy, for Sue became one aspect of the means by which professionals can make either a positive or a negative impact on people's lives. Later on it found expression in the aspiration that *clients are treated as well or better than staff—and that doesn't mean you treat your staff badly, it just means that your client areas need to be as good as your staff areas.* Power can be used to communicate respect for service users, or it can be used to separate and control. For Sue the former is good practice and the latter is a misuse of power.

One of the main responsibilities that follow from professional power is that of accountability. This can take different forms. In one example Sue talks about her sense that there are possible issues that were not fully addressed for a young Indigenous woman who had given up her baby for adoption. So when, many years later, Sue found herself working with Indigenous colleagues on a conference to examine the *Bringing Them Home* report into the Stolen Generation she continued to feel a sense of responsibility to be accountable for past practices, irrespective of whether her own actions could be regarded as good or bad in terms of the welfare of the child, because *for me the line between child protection and Stolen Generation, even as late as the early seventies, was still very blurred*. More broadly, this approach to responsibility and accountability can be seen in Sue's view that technical language should be avoided as much as possible. Accountability can only be achieved when there is clear communication between professionals and service users, so that professionals should *privilege plain language and the capacity to engage people ... rather than use exclusionary language which would give [professionals] more power*. The question this poses for social workers is: *How can you have all this knowledge and understanding and espouse self-determination and inclusion and then function exactly the opposite to that?*

This view leads to a position where the meaning of professionalism is found in service. There is a strong similarity between Sue's position and that articulated by Sercombe (2010, p. 10) that professionals "do not provide a service, we serve". This can be seen in many aspects of Sue's career, in which she appears to have focused on what was beneficial for service users or for a service such as Jenny House women's refuge in Newcastle, rather than what was easier for herself. Indeed, she is critical of what she sees as a different type of professionalism in social work where colleagues are either so focused on processes that they forget to attend to outcomes, or in which there appears to be a *lack of curiosity and the lack of initiative to find solutions beyond those that are ordained or acquired ... I see people critique policy but then not go on to the next stage*. Such an approach is not necessarily easy, however, as it requires commitment and also may involve compromise of the kind that can be seen in Sue's work with a government in the organisation of the CHOGM meeting, where that government may not match your own values.

Commitment and Resilience

Sue's life and career demonstrate several personal qualities that are crucial to understanding the way in which she has achieved the integration of personal and professional values. In particular, she demonstrates commitment and resilience in several ways. First, despite challenges and setbacks, she kept coming back to social work. In fact, with the exception of a short period working in a pest control agency in the 1970s, the whole of Sue's career has been in some aspect of social work. This has included casework, management of child welfare, teaching at both TAFE and universities and, most recently, the role of CEO in three large non-government organisations. Although Sue expresses some ambivalence about social work as a profession, throughout her adult life she has used it as a vehicle to pursue her values. In that sense it would appear that her commitment is to the underlying values rather than (always) to the profession. At the same time, these values appear to have formed a basis for her to be resilient in the face of challenges.

Possibly the biggest single challenge of this kind was in the death of her husband when she was aged 34, with two small children. Both in the way in which Sue faced this life crisis and in the way that she demonstrates learning from it and other somewhat less confronting experiences, she has developed insights that have contributed to her focus on helping others. These insights are formed empathically: while giving a concrete sense of what it is like to experience such deep loss, at the same time Sue's bereavement appears to have heightened her awareness that everyone deals with suffering in their own way.

In practical ways, the qualities of commitment and resilience are evident in how Sue has balanced professional and family life. This has involved sometimes making some very difficult choices that follow from a strong sense of responsibility as a parent and in caring for her own parents. On some occasions a change of job has been made in response to such family commitments, such as in moving back to Perth from Canberra in order to provide support for her parents. Yet at other times, finding ways to balance these different commitments has been possible, such as in the way Sue sought to be an active parent while at the same time undertaking a very demanding role in the disaster response work at Gracetown in the south of Western Australia.

Broader Values

Throughout her account of her life and professional career, Sue identifies key values that have provided a broad base for her thinking and practice. The first of these is that of non-maleficence, or seeking to do no harm. At one point, recounting an example of practice that had not produced a very good outcome, she exclaimed *what we do is harmful!* In several other parts of her story the theme of harm and the avoidance of harm as a primary social work goal is apparent. Sue sees this as a strong motivator for her own practice and also the decisions she has made about her career: *this do-no-harm thing is strong in me*. Again, she notes that as a social work teacher she told her students: *Don't do any harm and if you feel as though you're doing harm stand back*. In her current position with UnitingCare West, the Board and its chairperson overtly ask to be reassured that the organisation is not causing any harm. Sue's stance in advocating for homeless people in Perth during CHOGM came from an awareness that they were at risk of being harmed by the event, while on another occasion she was reluctant to have service users appear in media stories because of the harm that might follow for them personally. On the other side of the coin, Sue also refers to the value of beneficence or seeking to do good. Examples include practice in which a vulnerable child was protected while at the same time family relationships were maintained.

Second, although she does not refer to the concept overtly more than twice, Sue regards compassion as a quality that is very important for her. Here she is referring to a value that she finds expressed in her faith. The meaning of compassion that comes from her description of her work has parallels with Nussbaum's (2001) notion of an intelligent emotion in response to the serious plight experienced by another person, in which we also find a sense of shared humanity. This is most evident in the way in which Sue discusses her experience of being a service user immediately after the death of her husband, and its impact on her approach to working with service users throughout her following career. This awareness was evident before that critical event, but in her story it is given particular prominence by the pivotal significance of this experience.

Third, Sue greatly values competence or capability. Indeed her story from an early age demonstrates how important it is for her to evaluate herself and be seen by others as competent or capable. From this, she has then sought to emphasise other people's competencies and capabilities in her practice (and in her parenting). This is both an ethical position, in that it communicates the value that is placed on the humanity of others, and also a type of strengths approach [developed prior to that becoming a formal social work theory, cf. Saleebey (1996)].

Fourth, following on from the emphasis placed on competence, Sue clearly expresses humility. She is aware of her own limitations and of the importance of working as part of a team. In many places this is a balanced viewpoint, as it includes being able to express a sense of awareness of her own competence, for example in being a leader and being able to practise leadership that supports and enables others. At the same time there are also occasions on which humility risks becoming self-deprecation, such as when she describes herself as *this very ordinary person*. In particular, Sue is conscious of what she perceives as a lack of theoretical language in which to express policy and practice ideas—yet at the same time, as noted above, she values plain language, especially as a means to be inclusive of service users.

The final two broader points are expressions of what might be termed practical politics. The discussion above has already noted that Sue holds the view that social work may be prone to too much of a focus on process. She says:

> I think these days social work is vulnerable to only doing good process stuff. So for me the process has always only ever been about ensuring that you get good outcomes, respectful outcomes for your employer but good outcomes for people, and those sort of process things are not the end point. They are literally a way of being able to … make sure you know what the end point is of why you're engaged in somebody's life.

This sits alongside a conviction that being able to work within organisations and the politics of social welfare is vital to effective practice. Sue claims her motto is *follow the money* and she states, *I have a very strong view that you can't be an effective social worker unless you actually understand where the money is, who makes the decisions and how it transfers*. When social workers are willing to engage with material resources, and the compromises that can sometimes require, then there is greater potential for being able to set the agenda.

Conclusion

In 2014 "this very ordinary person" Sue Ash was recognised by the community in the award of the Order of Australia for her contribution to social work, for example in the social justice approach taken to looking after the interests of homeless and other disadvantaged people during CHOGM. While at times in her career Sue has felt ambivalent about social work, at this stage she says:

> I think over the last few years it's been great to own being a social worker and try and put something back into … our profession but also for the world actually seeing what social workers are capable of doing, to try and ensure that the social workers who we have got working now feel empowered and enabled to actually do some of that.

References

Nussbaum, M. (2001). *Upheavals of thought*. New York: Cambridge University Press.
Saleebey, D. (1996). The strengths perspective in social work: Extensions and cautions. *Social Work, 41*(3), 296–305.
Sercombe, H. (2010). *Youth work ethics*. London: Sage Publications.

Chapter 3
But You Can Push and Push and Push—Diana Batzias

Manohar Pawar

Diana Batzias was raised in country Victoria and educated in Adelaide. Immediately after her graduation from the University of Adelaide in 1963, she practised for a few years in London, working directly with immigrants and witnessing their lives. On her return, Diana worked with migrants and asylum seekers for about ten years at the Ecumenical Migration Centre in Melbourne. Building on that grassroots experience, she moved to the Victorian Department of Human Services in policy and program development and worked there for about 18 years, contributing significantly to the implementation of the Supported Accommodation Assistance Program (SAAP) and Youth Homeless Allowance, and initiatives arising from the Burdekin inquiry into youth homelessness.

Diana then assumed the role of Chief Executive Officer of the Melbourne Juvenile Justice Centre, formerly "Turana"—a custodial facility for young men—and was there for about nine years. During her term in office important institutional reforms were introduced under challenging circumstances.

Diana had a practice career of about 40 years, but after retirement she continued to offer her honorary/voluntary services to non-government organisations such as the Victorian Women's Trust and Whitelion, which supports young people returning to the community from custody. The analysis of her life story reveals her faith, commitment to core values and ability to fight with determination.

M. Pawar (✉)
Charles Sturt University, Wagga Wagga, Australia
e-mail: mpawar@csu.edu.au

M. Pawar et al. (eds.), *Empowering Social Workers*,
DOI 10.1007/978-981-10-3809-9_3

Early Life

Diana Batzias was born in 1943 in Adelaide. Her parents come from South Australia, her mother from the north of the state and her father from Adelaide. On his return from the Second World War, Diana's father farmed in Victoria and that is where Diana was brought up—within a small community in which most of the people were soldier settlers. She was the eldest of three children (two girls and a boy) and she grew up conscious of her parents' significant engagements with the community.

When Diana was young, she was baptised Anglican and confirmed at the cathedral in Adelaide, although she has not been a practising religious person. As her parents were not well off, she wore her mother's tennis dress to be confirmed. Diana said, *There wasn't a lot of money for fancy dresses or anything in those days, particularly because they were just starting to farm the property.*

Before marriage, Diana's mother trained as a children's nurse at the Adelaide Children's Hospital (now the Women's and Children's Hospital), but she did not keep her registration once she went to live in the country. However, she was able to make use of her nursing knowledge with local people. Diana's maternal grandmother started the first Country Women's Association (CWA) in South Australia and participated in the planting of trees to prevent soil erosion. With a background in such activities, Diana's mother encouraged interested women to come together, and she drove them to a nearby small town that had a CWA. The women participated in some social activities and developed cooking, sewing and other skills. Diana's mother also took little children in her Volkswagen bus to the nearest town so they could be vaccinated against polio and to access similar health services.

The property had a paddock very close to the school. They had a dairy cow and Diana was a good milker, while her mother made butter and many other things. Her mother also bought flour from Naracoorte and made all the bread and buns on a basic wood stove. Such were major regular chores at that time and it was *a good way of living in lot of ways*. However, many other children were not so fortunate. Some rode a horse to school and Diana remembers a family of six children who walked nearly ten kilometres to school every day. Their father was an alcoholic and the mother eventually left because of his alcoholism and violence. Diana's mother brought these children home with her own children for lunch and usually offered them a casserole or a roast because they always had meat at lunchtime.

Diana's father was the president of the fire brigade. He not only helped to establish the local fire brigade, but contributed to the formation of the regional body. Her parents also paid for building the community hall and were influential in making sure that the hall was used for community activities. Diana said, *My father was extremely generous*. The hall required that the local people raise money to keep it going with regular repairs and maintenance. It is still a meeting place for the small community.

Diana remembers that she was well taught at the local school and was encouraged to read at home. In those days there were no libraries, but her grandmother used to get a new book every month for her to read. Diana went to a boarding school in Hamilton for four years when she was eight years old and during that time visited home once a month. Her sister joined her as a boarder after two years.

As a 12-year-old child, Diana witnessed a bushfire at the farm and that experience has remained with her as one of the most tragic childhood experiences—one that she and her parents *never really got over.* Their house was damaged, though not badly. Of the 593 lambs, to be sold on the day of the fire, only three survived and because of the smell, the family could not eat meat for months. Diana's father went to help an older man and their truck was caught in the fire. A man died when he jumped from the truck to rescue his bull and, Diana said, *My father never forgave himself. He couldn't have done anything more to save him but it was very sad.* As telephone lines were defunct, her mother went down the road, about 16 km, to the next small village to inform the people there about the imminent fire and the need for preparation. No adult was home during the fire, and Diana felt responsible for her siblings and three children of another family that worked for Diana's parents. She put all of them in a big concrete tank and they used tyres to float on the water, and they remained there until the fire passed the house. Diana said:

> Looking after the kids in the tank was a big responsibility and I felt that responsibility because I was the oldest [12 years] of all the kids and I was the only older one left there. However, in the country you do what you can do even as a child.

Diana's mother accompanied an injured person to Naracoorte Hospital in the back of a truck, and they thought she was an Aboriginal as she looked so dirty due to bush-fire work. She finally convinced them that she was on the hospital committee. A couple of families had lost their houses in the fire and Diana's parents provided shelter to them in their workmen's cottages. To Diana all this was part of living in the community. The bushfire was *really a catastrophic time for my parents and they put a lot of work into fighting it, and then starting again in lots of ways.*

Move to Adelaide for Further Studies

When Diana was 12 years old she boarded at Walford Anglican school in Adelaide. She had an older cousin to keep an eye on her there. She lived with her grandparents in the last two years of school, which saved some money for her parents. After completing the schooling, Diana thought of doing law, but her age did not permit this as she was only 16. To be eligible she had to undertake one year of study at Adelaide University, and that year incorporated social sciences and arts subjects, including social economics. It was this exposure that helped Diana decide not to do law, but social work. It was thus a career turning point.

Diana said: *I know it [social work] was the right thing for me. I would never have been happy with that [law].*

But to her father, going to university was a waste of time and he was not in support of Diana doing social work, as he wanted her to do something useful like her mother had. In the end, her father was very happy and proud about Diana's studies at the university. She remembers that she was in the group of 15 bright students, and she relished the wideness of the course and did well, gaining a lot of distinctions. Her placements she remembers as fantastic; one was at the Queen Victoria Hospital and the other one was working in the field of carers' payments. Her final placement supervisor was fantastic. She encouraged Diana to work with her on developing a social service payment for carers. It was really a full-time job working with the supervisor, but it turned out to be a wonderful educational opportunity for Diana:

> Well I remember the fact that she allowed me to have a go even though I wasn't qualified … and the fact that she allowed me to participate in the early payment issues with the Commonwealth Government meant that already I was getting some experience of working with the Commonwealth Government. My experience came from observing my supervisor and from being permitted to become fully involved. She gave me the necessary information and then allowed me to have a go, which was something that not many supervisors would do. But she was at my shoulder should I need her …

Of the 15 students, only five graduated, and Diana was one of them.

Sailed off to Work in the UK—The First Social Worker Position

As a 21-year-old graduate, Diana sailed for England but, as was expected in those days, she got off the ship in Lisbon and made her way across Portugal and Spain, and through France, to England. She travelled by public bus, learning Spanish very quickly as a matter of necessity. On her second day in the UK she moved into a hospital almoner job for six months at Great Ormond Street Hospital for Children and then moved to Queen Charlotte Maternity Hospital in Hammersmith for another six months. At that time the almoners had to wear a white coat that had an almoner badge, but Diana said, *I must say, I didn't take kindly to being called an almoner.* She and a colleague from Chile preferred to call themselves social workers, because the term almoner carried the historical sense of giving something to the poor, and this did not appeal to Diana. Her work experience in the UK began her ongoing involvement in immigration work in lots of ways, because she met people from the Middle East, Trinidad, West Indies and elsewhere and was thrown into cross-cultural social work. She could not *believe that all the bus drivers were black.* Diana contrasted her life in the UK with her life in Australia as follows:

> I don't think I ever saw an Indigenous person until I was quite old in our own country; we had nothing at school about Indigenous people generally or our own Indigenous people. There were lots of problems with all of that area I think.

In the hospital Diana was *pretty horrified by children with deformity problems, often so severe that some of them probably did not have a very good future.* She was pop-eyed to see Arabic people coming into the hospital with "*a tea towel*" on their head to visit their children. Diana worked with West Indian immigrants who were having their first children and with Irish girls coming over to have their babies and have them adopted in the UK, and she said that *this was horrible to see.* Irrespective of whether the process was right or wrong, the Irish girls were generally anxious and sad, and this was a traumatic experience for Diana. She was also horrified to see the type of accommodation that the West Indian immigrants were living in, as she had not seen anything like that before. She thought that accommodation-related laws broke up families, meaning that even 10- or 12-year-old children could not stay with their mothers. Only one good thing she remembers was when Ringo Starr's baby, Zac, was born, their fans presented clothes and the family passed on all those presents to the almoners department, which in turn gave these clothes to West Indian babies, who looked beautiful in them.

After three and half years experience in the UK, including travel, Diana sailed back to Australia. She made money working at a little bar on the Greek ship. In the ship she observed British and Yugoslavian migrants on their way to Australia, and their hopes and naivety about their settlement prospects in Australia. The British spent most of the money they were given for the ship on alcohol and tobacco. The Yugoslavs were not able to speak English, so Diana contributed to the English classes that were held on the ship.

Return to Australia and Social Work Practice

Finding Adelaide a bit small after Europe, Diana applied for two jobs in Melbourne—as a social worker at the Alfred Hospital and with the Immigration Department. The Immigration position came through first and she chose to work with them, in part because of her exposure to immigrants on board ship from the UK. That experience had fascinated her, especially the naivety of British immigrants in regard to their settlement in Australia and their decision to return to the UK after a couple of weeks. Diana said: *I don't ever remember thinking I want to be a medical social worker for ever. I saw these people coming and wanted to be part of the community looking after them.*

While in the Immigration Department, Diana did some direct work with immigrants from England, Yugoslavia and elsewhere. At that time the economy was in a downturn, and many migrants with trade skills sought work in NSW, while some thought of returning to the UK due to the difference between their expectations and experiences and their isolation. Diana said, *You don't realise how important family members might be until you get away from the family.* In addition to her work at the Immigration Department, she served on the management committee of the Ecumenical Migration Centre (EMC). As she was very much attracted to the EMC's community relations, education and social-action work, Diana eventually became a staff member there.

At the EMC, Diana worked with immigrants from Turkey, Yugoslavia, Timor-Leste, Greece, Italy and Vietnam. She recollects that the work was mostly directly helping immigrants to settle in Australia, along with community work establishing basic services and lobbying for government services such as English language classes and child care. The case-work practice involved bringing/connecting family members and many *very practical things in lots of ways*. Diana also worked a lot with Greek women who came to Australia to marry, and with those who became single parents. She contributed to policy and program work at the EMC.

During the Whitlam era, the agency was successful in getting grants to provide specialised and much-needed services such as English classes, translation services and the establishment of small-scale facilities. The staff worked in the first high-rise flats built by the Victorian Government's Housing Commission in Richmond, and closely with the community health centre established opposite them. Interpreter services were an important issue at the time and practical approaches were developed to deal with language needs. All this intense work was done with the agency's meagre income. The EMC operated as a collective, meaning that all staff received the same income and, at that time, without any superannuation or other benefits.

From direct practice and community work Diana moved to policy and program work when she accepted another position within the Immigration Department. Among other things, she was responsible for setting up the translation service at the request of The Hon. Al Grassby, Federal Minister for Immigration from 1972 to 1974, and it was he who launched the service. Diana's direct work experience at the EMC helped her to appreciate the nature of the needs for translation and interpreter services. She noted the existence of privatised and unreliable translation services provided by some individuals, where issues related to trust and confidentiality were at stake. Diana was significantly involved in the practical setting up of the translation and interpreter scheme in terms of the setting of standards and the preparation of workers, along with the provision of free access to these services by those who needed them. Diana said: *It was a fantastic service. Before this, all such services had been private and people had had to pay. The new service meant that people could now get free service and this was essential.*

Diana is considered to be one of the pioneers who contributed to establishing this free translation service for immigrants across Australia. She frequently visited Canberra for meetings related to carer allowances, youth allowances, and she had very good staff members who had strong backgrounds and who could discuss the policies and programs that they would like to see happen. Diana said: *We were not always successful but you can push and push and push and you'd be pleased to get 50 per cent or less of what you asked for. But there were also often times when you were successful.*

Diana believes *It's important to work out who the big players are and you need to get them on side, no doubt about that.* For her, equally important was the involvement and support of the community outside the government. She said:

> We went to Canberra several times to negotiate community involvement and the first immigrant women's services came out of that, as did the services for refugees, placements for the homeless among both older people and young people, which was a program that was desperately needed and I'm sure is still needed. I found that work really rewarding.

During the 1980s, Diana was the Director of the Community Support Program in Victoria. Although she did not develop this program, she was responsible for implementing it, with a multi-million-dollar budget. By negotiating between federal and state governments, Diana significantly contributed to establishing women's refuges and related services. She was responsible for the development and operation of Neighbourhood Houses, the Supported Accommodation Assistance Program (SAAP) and the Home and Community Care (HACC) program under which several crucial services were provided to the community. A colleague who worked for one of these commented on Diana's leadership as follows:

> Our paths first crossed in the late 80s—and very distantly—but the impact of her leadership was profound. The SAAP unit were visionary people who demonstrated confidence, autonomy and loyalty—all roads leading to Diana Batzias.

Diana also played a significant role in expanding state-wide Neighbourhood Houses, which were geared towards mutual support, community development and personal growth opportunities for women and children by providing funding, but communities were expected to manage them themselves. With a couple of bright women, Diana successfully developed a budget item for the state-level election to reduce water and electricity bills for people who did not have adequate income.

She continued to work in the Community Services, Victoria, although she experienced a difficult relationship with a secretary who was a very brilliant and strong man, but Diana was not on his right side. Later, he came to regard Diana well. It appears that he threw Diana into a tough situation by asking her to head the Juvenile Justice Centre (JJC), which was experiencing strikes and staffing issues, with a promise that he would provide the necessary support. Contrary to this head's anticipation, Diana embraced the job, although she did not receive support as promised to run the centre. However, she was very sad when this person passed away.

Then, for about nine years, Diana headed the JJC and introduced significant reforms for the welfare and rehabilitation of detained young people. Before any such reforms, the task given was to resolve the strike by staff members. There were only two women employees in the JJC. Diana engaged another woman as the unit manager, but that woman left within a few weeks, feeling that it was not a place for her, as the *blokes were terrible to her*, although she continues to be a good friend of Diana's. It was difficult for the male staff to accept a female head, and they generally thought that the JJC was not a place for female staff members. During the strike, Diana mobilised volunteers from Child Protection, the Salvation Army and various other organisations, who looked after the young people. Also a lot of the young people were released home with a plan to bring them back when the strike was over.

Diana began conversations with the union people in their accustomed style, discussed the new laws introduced by Premier Jeff Kennett's government and generally tried to pacify them. Remembering the situation, Diana said, *I was completely in the dark, in uncharted waters*. After the strike, the staff members she needed to get rid of were identified, although she still had a tough time with a few staff members. She was frightened to the extent that she thought of taking her telephone number off the public listing, but she was firm with the staff and had the support of the regional director. Eventually she was successful in removing them. Some other staff members left on their own to go to regional areas. The proportion of women employees was then increased up to 30%. Diana said, *families are made of men and women, so are social institutions and they're doing the same job but they do it differently, sufficiently for both to be useful*.

She directly intervened in children's fights and resolved them. She said, *I was never afraid of a kid the whole time I was there*. Some staff members' approaches were not conducive to children's wellbeing, as they wanted to drag them off and put them in isolation. By removing rorts and so freeing up resources, health teams and other programs were able to be introduced. Moreover, instead of leaving it to government architects, Diana and her colleague were heavily involved in preparing separate architectural designs for boys' and girls' centres, and finally they won this battle. To break the common institutionalisation of girls, they put them in community houses. The fares of Aboriginal parents were paid so they could visit their children.

For Diana the most difficult experiences in the JJC were two deaths of children in custody. As head of the centre she took responsibility for these sad incidents, which might have occurred due to lapses on the part of staff members on duty. Diana said, *You never get over the guilt of that*. Overall she said, *I was pretty proud of all we achieved I have to say, as were the women who worked with me*. After nine years, in 2009 Diana retired, exhausted by what had been a most demanding position.

It appears, however, that she retired only from the JJC, but not from the work. She undertook a short-term assignment with the Salvation Army, regarding improvement of their services to refugees and immigrants. In addition, Diana was the President of the Australian Board of International Social Service (ISS) for a number of years and retired from that position only last year, although she continues to be a member of the Board. Diana helped to establish a not-for-profit community service organisation, namely Whitelion, which *provides youth-focused gender and culturally specific services in several areas, which include mentoring, employment, specialist outreach support and education-based prevention programs* (http://www.whitelion.asn.au/). She has also supported in whatever ways she could the work of the Refugee Council of Australia. Diana is also actively involved in the Victorian Women's Trust, on its Board as well as a member of a small group of Board members who assess and assign grants to community groups. She continues to work for the welfare of the people and believes in lifting people up. She contributes to petitions and writes to ministers on issues that she thinks are important.

In her personal life, Diana was married to a Greek immigrant, and they had two boys, but after 16 years they separated. Although *in the interim it was a difficult time, with the coming along of three grandchildren everything is friendly now*, said Diana. As one son has to sleep after doing night shifts as a paramedic, on some days of the week Diana looks after her granddaughter, always pushing herself to do more.

Analysis of Qualities/Character

At the time of interview Diana was 71 years old, not keeping well and overcoming jet lag from an overseas trip. She kept pushing herself during the interview, warning that she was experiencing some memory loss and that, therefore, some of the facts and sequence of events in the narration may not be fully accurate. Throughout her life and career Diana has kept pushing and pushing and pushing herself. It is, therefore, interesting and useful to look at some of the qualities that have helped her accomplish what she has achieved by this pushing and pushing.

Commitment to Community

Throughout her life and career Diana's commitment to community has remained unshaken. Whether she worked in direct practice, overseas, on the ship, in policy-making and program delivery, in institutions, in not-for-profit-sector organisations, Diana usually looked at her work from a community perspective. She significantly contributed to creating communities for refugees and immigrants, women and children, and around institutions and organisations. For example, she was *very committed to the work that ISS does internationally*. Based on her practice, Diana said, *If you believe in community being important then you have to involve them on both sides*. She spoke about how, when she was working at the EMC, they conducted feisty meetings and intensely engaged the community members, even when, on one occasion, some of them gave boos, boos and boos to the minister who had suggested removing them from the current place of residence. Due to a very strong campaign, the community stayed where they were and the minister backed down. Whatever work she did, Diana often linked it to the community. In her early life it appears that she was greatly influenced by her parents, who were themselves significantly engaged in community activities. Diana said, *I got from my mother and my father a commitment to community and I guess that's always stayed with me*.

Charity and Love: Qualities Influenced by Religion and Faith

Religion and faith systems, if one believes in them, contribute to the development of values and character. Diana voluntarily said, *I'm a baptised Anglican, confirmed Anglican, but I'm not a practising one. However, I believe in the sorts of values that come through those sorts of places*. Some of those values are: being generous to and looking after neighbours and your family; practising charity in its best form; and not just giving second-hand clothes. Charity to her was supporting people who might not be able to support themselves, and she thinks that such values come from every religion. *It is about lifting people up from difficult situations, just as it is in the Bible*. Diana thinks that what she has always tried to do, both with her family and her interest in the community, come through that.

Sense of Social Justice and Fairness

It appears that from the very beginning Diana cultivated a strong sense of social justice and fairness. She said she *does not believe in the dripping down of resources to people down below*. It was important for her to develop an *understanding of other people's lesser opportunities*, which she was conscious of from her school days. Implicitly questioning one kind of charity, Diana asserted, *I must say I didn't take kindly to being called an almoner*. She was also quick to recognise the unreliable translator who *charged people heaps of money*. Diana did not approve of agencies providing second-hand underclothes and one jacket to three people. As a young graduate, when she was exposed to multicultural populations and issues in London, her response was: *I don't think I ever saw an Indigenous person until I was quite old in our own country; we had nothing at school about Indigenous people, our own people. There were lots of problems with all of that I think.*

It was horrible for her to see *Irish girls coming over to have their babies adopted*. This strong sense of social justice and fairness was translated through various services and programs that Diana was responsible for, both in government and non-government organisations.

Commitment to Gender Issues and Feminist Principles

A colleague who has worked with Diana stated that she has a strong commitment to feminist principles. Diana described a worker who designed a part of the building for girls in the JJC as fiercely feminist, but she herself did not claim to be such. However, her work seems to have been always explicitly about her commitment to gender issues and feminist principles. She was empathetic to Irish girls who came to London to deliver their babies; she also worked with Greek women who came to Australia to marry and became single parents; and she found a deep sense of reward when she played a role in establishing the first women's services and refuges for women. Through Neighbourhood Houses, an educational provision for women and children was also provided.

When she became head of the JJC, she found only two women on staff, but during her leadership Diana increased women staff members to 30%. She said, *families are made of men and women, so are social institutions. They're doing the same job but they do it differently, sufficiently to be useful*. Further, *all three of us were women and I have to say, I think, it changed some dynamics*. As an active member of the Victorian Women's Trust and its grant committee, Diana played a role in assessing and assigning $300,000 to attend to health and other issues of women and to raise awareness of women's rights among migrant women.

Diana clearly believes in financial independence and liberty for women. Through the trust's Rosie project, they are reaching out to young women (aged 12–18) in the country to make them aware of—and able to access—available services.

Loving/Enjoying One's Own Work

Enjoying work has connotations of satisfaction from work rather than doing it successfully; fulfilment and a meaningful life rather than a life of pleasure. An ability and human quality to love and enjoy what one does is vital for any profession, any practice and any work, but perhaps even more so in social work. Social work is a path often not full of roses. Every day, social workers deal with complex issues and needs, at whatever level they work. Do you every day look forward to going to work where clients present complex problems, are distressed and depressed, victimised, powerless both in terms of resources and circumstances, present demands that may appear unreasonable, and sometimes become angry, abusive or unco-operative? Often there are no clear solutions and predictable outcomes, at least in some areas and situations. Sometimes bureaucratic organisations are not supportive or function contrary to your own values. Dropping a career in law and deciding to go into social work was a turning point for Diana. Social work has offered her a lot of rich experiences. She said:

> I never wanted to do anything else because I've always loved my work, I guess. I feel not many people love their work all their life and I always have and I think it's about individuals and community and all those sorts of things which I've been privileged to be involved with. So there's nothing very scientific about it. I mean I could have taken much more senior jobs, I could have done a whole lot of other things but I got in a mode that I was happy in and felt I was making a difference.

Diana feels blessed to have had the education that enabled her to move into an area that she has enjoyed her whole life, and to work as a social worker in different arenas was to her a privilege. Diana said, *I would never have been happy with law.* Over 50 years passionate practice in social work in different capacities and arenas shows how heavily Diana was involved and how much she has loved and enjoyed her work: *I enjoy being part of organisations now that are still trying to make a difference in the policy/program areas.*

Protest, Fight and Push

Perhaps drawing on her own ethos and values, Diana portrays in her biographic interview a feature of protest, fight and push. This was evident throughout her work.

When she and her colleagues tried for new programs or services, Diana said, *We were not always successful but you can push and push and push and you'd be pleased to get 50% or less*. When they fought and pushed new building designs in the JJC, Diana said, *We won the battle I'd have to say*.

How Diana used or managed with this quality in government organisations would be an interesting question for further exploration. She described one of her colleagues as *wonderful, gutsy, fighting all the way*. Having initiated so many reforms in the JJC, and looking at the current juvenile justice system, Diana said: *Now the juvenile justice system is a jail—it's just awful what's happened. You work yourself around the positives and then they all disappear with the next government. It's really horrible*.

Reacting to the refugee and asylum-seeker policy, Diana's protest comes in these words: *There are some people in that government I would like to put on Manus Island themselves permanently. I won't name them but it's a sad time really because we were known as very generous takers of immigrants as a country*.

Diana often agrees with some of the big petitions that are being put up and sometimes writes to ministers about them. They are in relation to children's deaths or abuse in custody, women's issues and lack of health facilities. Diana is certainly maintaining the tempo of protest, fight and push.

Taking the Initiative to Establish New Programs and Services

Flowing from her commitment to the community, and by identifying needs in communities and issues related to meeting those needs, Diana took the initiative in establishing various programs and services. She was one of the trail blazers in establishing interpreter and translation services in the Department of Immigration. Other programs and services she helped to initiate include child-care centres; English language classes; women's services and refuges for women; education for women and children through Neighbourhood Houses; assessing and assigning grants; building a new Juvenile Justice Centre; facilitating parents' visits to inmates; reducing payments for essential services by the poor; creating a not-for-profit organisation, Whitelion; and contributing to the implementation of the newly initiated SAAP and HAAC programs. These and similar programs and services appeared ahead of their time. Many of these initiatives also required pushing hard and Diana tirelessly pushed for them, but she also found setting up such programs and services really rewarding.

Courage and Fear

From riding horses in her childhood to removing rorts in the JJC, the qualities of courage, confidence and determination stand out clearly in the life story of Diana.

Facing the bushfire as a young child, sailing overseas as a young adult, working in a new cultural context, taking initiatives in the unknown territories—some across the state—taking charge of the JJC when it was on strike, successfully dealing with the union matter, removing employees, facing deaths in custody and the Coroners Court, all call for courage, confidence and determination. Diana's work clearly demonstrated these qualities.

Equally, how Diana dealt with an opposite quality—fear—is insightful and perhaps instructive. Diana described how fearful she was:

> I was in the dark, I really was in the dark. It's amazing that the place didn't fall apart. Or that would have been quite good in some ways but it was not—when I look back on it I don't know how it survived or I survived, quite frankly. You just had to do what you had to do.
>
> I was frightened to even have my phone number in the phone book but …

Diana said she started smoking again because union persons were smoking; she started talking with them and reading the *Herald Sun* newspaper and began discussing new laws initiated by the government. She had to sort of pacify them. Although it took a long time, by gaining the support of the regional head, eventually Diana got firm with these employees and they left.

Diana put herself in the midst of children's fights and just changed the situation by being there. She said, *I didn't drag them off the floor or anything, I talked to them—talked to them, not bullied them. I was confident that I could do it, but I didn't see any other way. But it was a risk, it was a big risk.*

It appears that Diana was in perpetual motion around crisis. However, she was not able to get over the sense of guilt that came with two deaths in custody.

In other contexts, Diana described how a couple of social workers were gutsy women. These and similar experiences testify to Diana's own courage, confidence and determination, and her ability to overcome fear.

Quietly Unorthodox

A colleague described Diana as "quietly unorthodox". Diana's actions in many respects show her capacity to be unconventional or nonconformist in a constructive way. It is particularly challenging to do this in government organisations, where Diana worked for most of her career. Her unorthodoxy was apparent in her statement, *We sent a lot of kids home because they needn't have been in there anyway*; in her programs such as translation services and the introduction of a travel allowance for Aboriginal parents to visit their children; in the reformed roster system; in dealing with unions and removing and recruiting staff members; in the different building designs for girls; and in putting a strong case relating to ISS in an international conference and becoming unpopular for it. Diana said, *You have to sometimes be very unpopular because everyone's been the same thing for so long* and argued in the conference as follows:

> If we (ISS Australia) are part of a conglomeration organisation then we need to know what's happening. We need to have opportunities for making change. We need to be accountable to each other in individual cases but also in our policies.

Perhaps this quality of unorthodoxy has helped Diana to initiate many new services and programs, and to raise questions and deal with complex and challenging situations.

Responsibility

Diana's biography shows that she is a willing taker of responsibility. During her early life and later, she assumed several significant responsibilities. She took responsibility for her younger sister in the boarding school, for children during the bushfire, in social-work field placements, and in many positions in government and non-government organisations.

When Diana was asked to head the JJC, she said it was her background that made her not want to say *I cannot do this job*, which shows her willingness to take responsibility, though it was a new operational job compared to her past policy and program position. Diana believed that *if you're the leading person, if you're the boss, you have to take and I took responsibility*. In regard to the two deaths in custody, although the two workers' security/protective role was there, as a boss Diana did not believe in putting it down to workers. She said:

> It's about my philosophy which goes back to my family and everything else. You've got to take responsibility and if you've got the big capital letters up there, you've got to take the stuff, so, I guess, I defended in some ways the staff even though on both occasions they were not doing what they were supposed to be.

Strong and Tough Person

Diana did not describe herself as a strong person, but a colleague who worked with her stated that Diana was *conceptually and personally tough*. Diana described her placement supervisor as a strong person in many ways, because she was the first Australian social worker to work in Papua New Guinea. Without being strong and tough Diana would not have embraced the tasks she performed in a range of challenging positions. In the biographic interview record these qualities were not well pronounced, but the practice evidence suggests that Diana was a strong and tough person.

Futuristic—Forward Thinking

Although Diana addressed in her work "here and now" situations, as many do, she was a futuristic and forward-thinking person. Many of her initiatives were well ahead of their time. Diana attributed the source of this forward-thinking quality to what she saw in others. When she worked on youth and carer allowances from the Commonwealth Government's social security system, she said, *There were some very forward-thinking people who were wanting to see support for people who did not have it, unlike what we are doing now*. From a futuristic perspective, Diana believed that *the young people are the future of the country and they should be the first people to be given opportunities*.

Industriousness

Undoubtedly Diana was a very hard-working person. She often worked beyond her office hours. She said, *I'd often have to go over in the middle of the night, across town, to work in the JJC*. Sometimes she was there at 10 o'clock at night writing the programs. Diana enthusiastically said: *there is never a time to rest in trying to improve things and trying to ensure that people know what is available to help them*. Diana identified herself this way: *I was a doer*.

Intellectual Virtues

The biographic interview data showed that Diana often valued the quality of being intelligent and diligent. She said, *I was taught very well*; *I was with a bunch of people who were pretty smart*; *I had a couple of bright women working with me*; *He was brilliant I'd have to say* and *One was a brilliant woman*. These remarks, while describing her own peers and colleagues, suggest that Diana had great intellectual capacity and that she valued that quality in others.

Appreciating Colleagues

Diana was appreciative of colleagues who worked for her. She said her colleagues in the EMC were feisty and gutsy. She said the staff members who worked for her were fantastic. Diana humbly admitted that another staff member who worked on the design of the building was much better than she was. She also said how bright women were working for her. How Diana adapted to another staff member was impressive: *A colleague was a night person; I was a morning person and so we actually both of us had to deal with that and often the colleague won*.

Generosity

The biographic interview suggested that Diana was a generous person. She perceived her father as a very generous person due to his support for and activities in the community. She also found Jewish women very generous. Diana donated some money to the Refugee Council of Australia, which is about the only group that is still agitating for a better deal for refugees. Diana laments that Australia was known at one time as a generous country for immigrants and refugees, but that it is now no more. She said that she would rather give money to the three organisations where she is a Board member than go and buy a new dress.

When she worked for the EMC she was paid almost nothing. It was a kind of collective; everybody got the same amount, no superannuation, nothing. Diana was conscious of giving back to the community. She said: *Well it's giving back I think. I see it as giving back because I feel I was blessed with a working life where I was paid to (pause) ... and I was paid not badly as a public servant for all that time ...*

Conclusion

Diana has relentlessly pushed herself, lifting people up in keeping with her own values and beliefs, and leaving an inspiring track. It may be apt to conclude her life story, qualities and character by quoting a remark by a work colleague:

> I see her, in Donna Jagg's (a social worker) words, as a wilful and passionate woman having a very rigorous value base with a strong commitment to social justice and feminist principles—but tempered by a diplomacy that is almost seductive, a great policy head and strategic savvy. She is conceptually and personally tough, with a resilience born of extraordinary compassion and a practicality that is potent, given that she does not take her eye off the big picture. Quietly unorthodox, she is a woman of enormous bravery.

References

Community Services Victoria Annual Report, 1987–1988. Retrieved November 12, 2014 from http://www.parliament.vic.gov.au/papers/govpub/VPARL1988-92No35.pdf

Whitelion. Retrieved November 12, 2014 from http://www.whitelion.asn.au/

Chapter 4
Empower People to Take Control of Their Own Lives—Tom Calma, AO

Andrew Alexandra and Manohar Pawar

Professor Tom Calma, AO, is an elder from the Kungarakan and Iwaidja tribal groups from the south-west Darwin region and the Cobourg Peninsula in the Northern Territory. Tom served about 45 years in the Australian public sector with a difference. Some of the notable positions he held in his service were the Aboriginal and Torres Strait Islander Social Justice Commissioner and Race Discrimination Commissioner[1] and he served as a senior Australian diplomat in India and Vietnam. Tom has dedicated his life to the cause of human rights and social justice, and empowerment of Aboriginal and Torres Strait Islander Australians. His outstanding contributions were officially recognised by honorary doctorates from Charles Darwin (2010), Curtin (2011) and Flinders (2014) universities, and he was made an Officer of the Order of Australia (AO) in June 2012 for distinguished service to the Indigenous community as an advocate for human rights and social justice, through contributions to government policy and reform, and to cross-cultural understanding.

Tom was named the ACT Australian of the Year in 2013, and in 2014 he was appointed Chancellor of the University of Canberra, the first Aboriginal person to become chancellor of an Australian university. In November 2014 Tom was awarded the Indigenous Allied Health Australia Lifetime Achievement Award in recognition of his lifelong dedication to improving the lives of Aboriginal Australians.[2]

[1]See https://www.humanrights.gov.au/news/media-releases/commission-welcomes-appointment-new-aboriginal-and-torres-strait-islander-social.

[2]http://iaha.com.au/events/2014-indigenous-allied-health-awards/ and http://www.canberra.edu.au/about-uc/media/monitor/2014/february/20-new-chancellor.

A. Alexandra (✉)
University of Melbourne, Melbourne, Australia
e-mail: a.alexandra@unimelb.edu.au

M. Pawar
Charles Sturt University, Wagga Wagga, Australia
e-mail: mpawar@csu.edu.au

M. Pawar et al. (eds.), *Empowering Social Workers*,
DOI 10.1007/978-981-10-3809-9_4

Tom was appointed a professor at the University of Sydney Medical School from 1 January 2015, to perform the role of Chair and Patron of the Poche Indigenous Health Network.[3]

In October 2015 Tom was awarded one of four Inaugural University of South Australia Alumni Awards for his service to society and in November of that year was awarded the Public Health Association of Australia's pre-eminent Sidney Sax Public Health Medal for notable contribution to the protection and promotion of public health, advancing community awareness of public health measures and advancing the ideals and practice of equity in the provision of health care.[4]

On 30 June 2016 in Canberra the Honourable John Berry, Ambassador of the United States of America to Australia, presented Tom with a US flag that was flown over the Martin Luther King Junior Memorial in Washington, DC, in recognition of his "leadership in promoting equality, social tolerance and youth advancement".[5]

In October 2016 Tom was appointed the foundation Chair of the Atlantic Fellows for Social Equity program, a US philanthropic and government-funded leadership collaboration hosted by the University of Melbourne.[6]

Analysis of his life and practice shows inspirational contributions and qualities.

Childhood and Education

Tom was born in 1953, spending the first three years of his life in Adelaide River among his mother's Kungarakan people. In Adelaide River Tom's father worked for the government, first as a road worker, then as a truck driver. When Tom was three the family made the approximately 100 km trip to Darwin, the home town of his father, who was a member of the Iwaidja people, whose lands stretch to the north-east of Darwin. That move allowed Tom's father to take up a position as a leading hand and to further his education at night school, after leaving school at the age of 14. He rose to become a senior public servant, supervising all the civil construction in the Darwin area, with a workforce of about 80 people, half of whom were Aboriginal.

Tom's involvement in the life of his parents' communities and his Darwin childhood were both fundamental to the sense of self and the values that have informed his professional and personal life:

[3]http://pochehealth.edu.au.

[4]http://w3.unisa.edu.au/alumni/AlumniAwards/Alumni-awards.asp and https://www.google.com.au/?gws_rd=ssl#q=Sidney+Sax+Public+Health+Medal+%2B+Tom.

[5]https://au.usembassy.gov/ambassador-berrys-remarks-u-s-independence-day-canberra-2016/.

[6]http://www.atlanticphilanthropies.org/news/university-of-melbourne-to-lead-20-year-leadership-program-to-tackle-social-inequality.

the background of connection with the land, the stories and relationships with country with Warai people are important because it does really address the core of my beliefs and my identity as an Aboriginal person and has influenced a lot of the why I do things and also the way I do things.

The Darwin Tom grew up in was in important respects atypical of an Australian town of its era. It was then relatively small—with a population of between 20,000 and 30,000—but also strikingly and unusually multicultural, with significant groups of Chinese, Filipino, Italian, Greek and Eastern European extraction, as well as Anglo-Celtic and Aboriginal groups. The interaction of members of these different ethnic groups in common activities such as sports fostered a broadly tolerant and respectful culture, in which Tom was immersed. He was also struck by the solidarity and communal orientation of the various ethnic groups—notably the Italians and Chinese—and their ability to work together to produce desired changes. For Tom, these attitudes were similar to those which inhered in Aboriginal culture, although Aboriginals were held back from effective group action at the time by a range of economic and social factors.

Tom and his three sisters lived a stable, if modest, existence with their parents in Darwin. They were among the first Aboriginal families to move into the suburbs, into a government-owned house, which they subsequently purchased when Tom was in his teens. Tom's father had ongoing paid employment, while his mother mainly looked after the family. Though they never went without, they had little to spare, with Tom recalling that he wore cheap nylon shirts to school, unlike many of his classmates who wore cotton, and the family lived from pay cheque to pay cheque, supplementing their income with the products of their hunting and fishing expeditions. They sold some of their catch, they consumed some themselves and they shared some with others.

The proximity of his mother's country allowed Tom to spend a good deal of time there. He speaks warmly of his childhood experiences among his extended family—fishing and hunting, as well as playing cards and storytelling—and of the sharing and mutual support that helped instil his desire to help others and influenced his future choice of career.

Unusually for Indigenous people in that period, Tom and his sisters all completed secondary schooling. Tom's academic results were mixed, but he was a keen sportsman, particularly in Australian Rules football and water polo, and he occupied a number of positions of authority at school, including being a member of the student representative council, captain of sporting teams, and a prefect and deputy head prefect. The position of head prefect was decided by a vote among the students. Tom reports that there was a strong belief in the school community that he had in fact won the vote. Nevertheless, and despite his de facto leadership of the student body, the school authorities decided not to appoint him as head prefect, supposedly so that he would not be distracted from his studies. According to Tom: *That, I guess, was my first real experience of discriminatory practice—a practice that, at the time, was seen as perfectly acceptable.*

While Tom's childhood was happy and he suffered little from direct racial discrimination, his experiences were inevitably coloured by the problems endemic to the Indigenous community, in particular alcohol abuse, with its corollaries of domestic violence, poverty and ill-health. Those problems in turn reflected the structural disadvantages borne by the Indigenous community. The Northern Territory has long had the greatest ratio of Indigenous to non-Indigenous residents of any of the Australian states or territories. While this has helped Indigenous Territorians preserve a relatively robust cultural tradition and given them more political influence than elsewhere in Australia, it has not prevented them from experiencing the dispossession and concomitant deprivation consequent on European colonisation. Tom notes, for example, that *when I was born in some missions it was reported that 200 in 1000 of our babies were dying before they even reached the tender age of one.*[7]

Tom's mother's family lived on their ancestral country, so many of the family did not suffer the disassociation from country that had such a devastating effect on many Aboriginals. Nevertheless, in accordance with the prevailing assimilationist philosophy, they were actively discouraged from using their language and practising their culture, as indeed were Tom and his contemporaries. One of the most destructive forms that philosophy took was the policy of "forced removal" of Aboriginal children, particularly of racially mixed background, from their families and their country. Though Tom's parents were spared, two of his mother's sisters and her brother, and his father's sisters, were forcibly removed, as was his mother's mother. A number of the Indigenous students at the high school Tom attended, and whom he knew, had also been forcibly removed, and lived in the Retta Dixon residential home in Darwin. Aboriginal people were also largely economically disempowered: for example, it was common until well into the 1970s for Aboriginal workers in the Northern Territory, especially in the pastoral industry, where most of them were employed, to be paid mainly or totally "in kind"—by food, tobacco and clothing.

Tom had first-hand experience of the situation of pastoral workers, going with his aunt to cattle stations to carry their rations. While there he also experienced the racism that was entrenched in the pastoral industry, seeing, for example, a bullock being shot for food, with all the desirable cuts going to the (European) management, and the rest being left for the Aboriginal workers. In Darwin, many Aboriginals, including a number of Tom's cousins on his father's side, lived in tin sheds in an area known as 118. Tom recalls classmates who lived in this area coming to school not wearing a school uniform and without lunch.

The centrality of kinship to Aboriginal culture meant that from an early age Tom was part of a network of mutual assistance. The relative good fortune of his immediate family meant that they were well placed to provide help, and his father in particular emphasised to his children the importance of education both for their own security, and also to give them the means to help others. Tom acknowledges the importance of the sharing ethos with which he was imbued in his decision

[7]Tom Calma http://www.humanrights.gov.au/news/speeches/people-power-force-country-celebrating-5th-anniversary-close-gap-campaign-aboriginal.

to become a social worker. He also came to realise the limitations of trying to deal with the problems he had encountered simply by assisting individuals in their immediate needs, a realisation that was enhanced and provided with practical outlets through the skills of group work, community development and social process change that his social work studies provided.

Career

Tom completed his secondary schooling in 1971, with no thought, or opportunity, of tertiary study. For about five years (1972–1976) Tom undertook mainly office administrative positions (clerical assistant 1–3 and clerk 4 levels) with the Department of Housing and Construction. By 1976 Tom had decided that he wanted to work in a job where he could help others and started to seek out opportunities for further studies that would enable him to do so. He applied for, and was accepted into, a recently established Community Development and Social Work course, in a program called the Aboriginal Task Force, at the South Australian Institute of Technology (SAIT), which was exclusively for Aboriginal and Torres Strait Islanders. During 1977–1978, studying and living in Adelaide broadened Tom's horizons, including his getting to know fellow Aboriginal and Torres Straits Islander students from around Australia, as well as mixing with non-Indigenous students, one of whom he married. He remembers his two years at SAIT fondly: he and his wife still remain friendly with other couples they met there, and he is now the inaugural Patron of the Indigenous Alumni (Deadly Alumni) for the University of South Australia (the successor institution to SAIT).

While Tom would have liked to continue his studies, in 1979 he returned to Darwin, to be with his dying father. He immediately found a way of applying his social work training, becoming an Aboriginal Vocational Officer and working with remote Aboriginal communities to give them access to government services, enhance employment opportunities and provide training. He worked with the communities of Gunbalunya (also known as Oenpelli), Warruwi (Goulburn Island), Minjalang (Croker Island), and on the Tiwi Islands. In this position he was able to apply the empowerment and community development approach that he had learned at SAIT, an experience that both convinced him of the value of that approach and later caused him to lament the lack of consistency and persistence in government policies supposed to assist Indigenous groups.

Within a year of graduating, Tom became instrumental in the creation of a program of studies in Darwin similar to the Aboriginal Task Force in Adelaide, specifically for Aboriginal students. He chaired a course development group, comprising concerned Aboriginal citizens working with Dr. Mark de Graaf, an anthropologist who lectured at Darwin Community College. After funding was secured for a Certificate in General Studies course at pre-tertiary level, to commence in 1980 with an initial intake of 25 students, Tom also chaired the course management committee to develop curriculum and further courses. He was subsequently invited to apply for the position of counsellor for students in the course: once in the position he also undertook teaching duties, including in maths and Aboriginal studies, as Tom explains, *bringing an Aboriginal perspective to Aboriginal studies*. Tom in effect became the understudy of de Graaf, the course co-ordinator, who was committed to the taskforce being run by Indigenous people: at the end of the first year de Graaf made way for Tom, who became co-ordinator of the program and senior lecturer in 1981. The program expanded to become a department, initially within the School of Social Work, eventually offering five full-time courses, including a foundation program leading on to tertiary studies, with close to 300 students enrolled.

The program marked a significant development in Aboriginal education in the Northern Territory. It was important, of course, in providing what Tom describes as a *second chance at education* for so many young Aboriginal and Torres Strait Islander people. It was also noteworthy in being driven by Indigenous people: Tom's deputy and co-developer was Wendy Ludwig, a Kungarakan woman; and Peg Havnen and Norman Fry, also Indigenous Territorians, occupied senior teaching roles and both subsequently became co-ordinators of the program. Tom believes that his social work and community development training were important both in informing the content of the curriculum of the program as well as in giving him the skills to generate broad support for the establishment of a program of this sort.

While working at Darwin Community College Tom and some of his colleagues became interested in the possible impact of the Aussat satellite. The launch of the satellite, scheduled for 1985, would make mass communication available to remote communities for the first time. In 1984 Tom was awarded an Aboriginal Overseas Study Award to investigate the impacts of satellite communication on language, culture and social behaviour and its role in the provision of distance education to Indigenous and remote communities. He travelled to Suva, Fiji and Hawaii, looking at tertiary education delivery to people in the Pacific; to the Open University in the United Kingdom; to Wales to look at the program for the revival of the Welsh language; and to the US and Canada. Tom wrote a study based on his findings but, as it transpired, a Senate Committee headed by Professor Eric Wilmot was examining these issues at the same time and had sent a working party to many of the places Tom had visited, and it was the recommendations of the committee, broadly similar to those of Tom's study, which formed the basis of government policy. Though Tom's trip had no immediate practical effect, it provided a foundation for his future work in international education, and influenced his views on the importance of bilingual education for Indigenous groups.

While Tom was an academic he had been on extended leave from the Commonwealth Public Service: in 1986 he was invited to rejoin as a director in charge of Indigenous employment. From 1986 until 1992 he occupied a range of positions in the area of employment, education and training and rose to become Director of Employment and Training (in the Commonwealth Department of Employment, Education and Training), and Acting State Director. Through his association with senior non-Indigenous public servants he became increasingly interested in finding work beyond the Northern Territory. He applied unsuccessfully for a UNESCO counsellor position in Paris, which he learnt about from the Secretary of Education in the Northern Territory, Geoff Spring, who was also the Australian representative on UNESCO in Paris. Around the same time he was encouraged by Greg Taylor, the Secretary of the Department of Employment, Education, Training and Youth Affairs (where Tom was then working), to participate in a trial program to bring senior state and territory based public servants to Canberra to develop their skills. In 1992, Tom and his family—by then including two children, shortly to be joined by a third—moved to Canberra.

While Tom and his wife had envisaged their move from Darwin as temporary, once in Canberra the employment opportunities open to them made them decide to settle there. Soon after arriving, Tom and a number of other Indigenous public servants decided that they should institute an Indigenous support program within the department and sought funding from Derek Volker, then Secretary of the Department of Employment, Education and Training. Volker backed the formation of the Aboriginal and Torres Strait Islander Network (ATSINet), which subsequently guided the establishment of the Indigenous Australian Public Service Employees Network (IAPSEN), operating across the whole Commonwealth Public Service; he also offered Tom a job as his executive officer.

In the early 1990s the Australian government, starting to see the potential for education to become a major export market, created five diplomatic positions, in Indonesia, Malaysia, Thailand, Vietnam and India. The aim was not just to encourage foreign students to come to Australia, but also to develop relationships with host-country governments and to assist them in the development of their own education systems. Tom secured the India posting, starting work on 1 January 1995 as an Education and Training Counsellor, tasked with establishing education offices in New Delhi and Mumbai. In that role he worked with all sectors of education, from primary to tertiary, to facilitate collaboration between Australian and Indian institutions and to support the recruitment of fee-paying students. While in India he also established offices in Pakistan, Nepal and Sri Lanka, coming to oversee the largest region of any counsellor.

Tom's work as an Education and Training Counsellor involved negotiations with a range of stakeholders—not only foreign governments, educational institutions and potential students, but also student recruiting agents and Australian officials in embassies and high commissions, including the Department of Immigration, who had to develop criteria for determining who would be found to be a bona fide student to be admitted into Australia. One of Tom's lasting achievements was the establishment in 1996 of an Agents' Association known as AAERI (Association of Australian Education Representatives in India). In August 2016 AAERI celebrated its 20th anniversary and the Minister for Education, the Honourable Simon Birmingham, MP, described AAERI as "a valued partner in the Australian Government's efforts to strengthen our international education offerings".[8]

[8]https://www.youtube.com/watch?v=LFHBMi7_9Fw&feature=share.

Recruiting agents were required to register with the association and abide by its code of ethical practices and good governance conduct.

Reflecting on his achievements in India—and later, in a similar role in Vietnam—Tom attributed his ability to communicate with a wide range of people to his training in public speaking as a school prefect, which he had furthered through his social work and teaching experiences. He also stressed the importance of his social work background, and in particular his knowledge of community development in allowing him to see the bigger picture and find ways of communicating that vision to others and help them to see how they could be part of it.

In 1998 Tom moved to Vietnam, to run the education offices there. By this time the Education and Training Counsellor scheme had expanded into Europe and America and the relationship with Australian education institutions was being put on a commercial footing: the services that had previously been provided free were now charged for. This involved a major change in the mindset on both sides of the relationship, as the details of the new commercial arrangements were worked out. Despite his lack of commercial experience, Tom proved adept at generating revenue under the new system, to the extent that the department estimated that in 1999–2000 the Vietnam office accounted for about a third of the global income of the counsellor network. One of the important sources of that revenue was Atlantic Philanthropy, an American-based philanthropic group that wanted to do work in Vietnam and had sought Tom's support. As an Australian diplomat he could only work with Australian institutions, but he entered into an arrangement whereby Atlantic Philanthropy provided funds to Australian education institutions (notably the University of Queensland) to provide scholarships to Vietnamese students, conditional on Tom being engaged to operate on the institutions' behalf in Vietnam, including recruitment, assessment and quality control.

While in Vietnam Tom also undertook market research for the Royal Melbourne Institute of Technology (RMIT) to determine the feasibility of their establishing a presence in Vietnam. On the basis of Tom's findings, and again with Atlantic Philanthropy support, RMIT entered into a twinning agreement with a local institution and opened an office in Ho Chi Minh City. This was the beginning of what has become a substantial RMIT presence in Vietnam, with a number of campuses and offices across the country. More broadly, Tom helped make Vietnam a more attractive place for foreign education institutions, working with the Australian Ambassador, Michael Mann, to persuade the Vietnamese Government to change their Education Act, which restricted the presence of foreign institutions in Vietnam and prohibited repatriation of moneys earned there.

Tom's second term as Education and Training Counsellor finished in 2002. Obliged by departmental policy to return to Australia, he briefly worked in Indigenous Affairs, reviewing education programs, before becoming senior adviser to Philip Ruddock, then Minister for Immigration and Indigenous Affairs, thereby gaining exposure to, and experience in, the workings of Parliament. When Ruddock became Attorney-General Tom returned to the Public Service to run the Community Development and Education Branch in the Aboriginal and Torres Strait

Islander Services (ATSIS), the recently created administrative arm of the Aboriginal and Torres Strait Islander Commission (ATSIC).

About a year after his return to Australia, Tom won the job of Aboriginal and Torres Strait Islander Social Justice Commissioner with the Human Rights and Equal Opportunity Commission (as it was then called), the government-funded body that oversees the application of federal legislation in the areas of human rights, anti-discrimination, social justice and privacy, and at the same time was appointed the Race Discrimination Commissioner, taking up these positions in mid-2004. He served as the Social Justice Commissioner until 2010 and as the Race Discrimination Commissioner until 2009. The position of the Aboriginal and Torres Strait Islander Social Justice Commissioner was created in 1992: its immediate impetus was the shocking findings of the Royal Commission into Aboriginal Deaths in Custody and the National Inquiry into Racist Violence; more broadly, it was a response to the extreme and ongoing social and economic disadvantage faced by Indigenous Australians. The commissioner's role includes reviewing the impact of laws and policies on Indigenous peoples, reporting on Indigenous social justice and native title issues and promoting an Indigenous perspective on issues. The Social Justice Commissioner also monitors the enjoyment of human rights by Indigenous Australians.

As Social Justice Commissioner, Tom was mandated to report to Parliament annually on issues affecting Aboriginal and Torres Strait Islander communities and peoples, including the impact of government policies and practices. In Tom's first full report[9] in 2005, he focused on Indigenous health through the lens of human rights, setting the theme for his ongoing work in this area. The report highlighted the fact that the life expectancy of Aboriginal and Torres Strait Islander people was 17 years less than that of the general population; the life expectancy of Aboriginal and Torres Strait Islanders was the same as that of people living in rural Bangladesh. By contrast, in other relevantly similar settler societies such as New Zealand, Canada and the US, the life expectancy gap was around six to seven years.

The right to health is one of the "core provisions" of the International Covenant on Economic, Social and Cultural Rights, to which Australia is a party. Tom drew on research highlighting the emerging discipline of social determinants of health—the associations between an individual's social and economic status and their health. Poverty is clearly associated with poor health, with poor education and literacy limiting the capacity of people to use health information; low income reducing access to health care services and medicines; overcrowded and run-down housing contributing to the spread of communicable disease; and smoking and other high-risk behaviours more common among lower socio-economic groups. Importantly, research has also shown that poorer people tend to have less financial and other forms of control over their lives, which can produce chronic stress, which is associated with a range of health problems: diseases of the circulatory system

[9]Tom Calma 'Social Justice Report' https://www.humanrights.gov.au/publications/social-justice-report-2005-home accessed 14/11/2014.

(notably heart disease), mental health problems, violence against women and other forms of community dysfunction.

In his report, Tom pointed to the relevance of another of the core provisions of the covenant, the "principle of progressive realisation", which recognises that while it may not be possible fully to achieve some rights in the short term, states (international term used to refer to sovereign governments) are required to take action, particularly legislative measures, which move in that direction. In light of this provision, Tom outlined a number of indicators of improvements in Indigenous health (such as reduction in infant mortality) and achievable targets to be met in specified time frames. While investment in primary health-care services was obviously fundamental in meeting such targets, as the research on the social determinants of health showed, such investment needed to be accompanied by initiatives to improve education, housing, employment and the like, with stress on active engagement of Indigenous communities in shaping and participating in such initiatives.

Implicit in the social determinants approach to Indigenous health was the need for a co-ordinated approach from all involved groups. Following the tabling of his report, Tom engaged with the major health peak bodies, both Indigenous and non-Indigenous, such as the Australian Medical Association, the Australian General Practice Network, and the National Aboriginal Community Control Health Organisations, as well as human rights organisations and other non-government bodies to develop a broad united coalition, with more than 40 members in total. The aim of the coalition was not to control the activities of its members, but rather to ensure that they would advocate with one voice to the government, the first time they had done so.[10] In April 2007 it launched the Close the Gap campaign,[11] organised by the National Aboriginal Community Controlled Health Organisation, Oxfam Australia and Australians for Native Title and Reconciliation, aiming to persuade governments around Australia to commit to closing the life expectancy gap within a generation. The campaign mobilised an estimated 140,000 Australians to write to politicians across the political divide.

Following the election of the new Labor federal government in November 2007, the Council of Australian Governments (COAG), representing federal, state and territory governments, made the desired commitment and agreed to be accountable for achieving it within the specific time frame of 2031. This commitment, known as the National Integrated Strategy for Closing the Gap, had targets that went beyond health and picked up some of the key social determinant challenges. In 2008, the Australian government and peak Indigenous health organisations signed the

[10]See file://www.Volumes/TSB%20USB%20DRV/Socialworkproject/What.%20is%20the%20history%20of%20Closing%20the%20gap%3F%20%C2%AB%20Key%20facts%20%C2%AB%20Closing%20the%20gap%20%C2%AB%20Australian%20Indigenous%20HealthInfoNet.html accessed 15/11/2014

[11]https://www.humanrights.gov.au/our-work/aboriginal-and-torres-strait-islander-social-justice/projects/close-gap-indigenous-health and https://www.oxfam.org.au/what-we-do/indigenous-australia/close-the-gap/.

Indigenous Health Equality Summit Statement of Intent, stating that they would "work together to achieve equality in health status and life expectancy between Aboriginal and Torres Strait Islander peoples and non-Indigenous Australians by the year 2030".[12] The Queensland, Victorian, Australian Capital Territory, Western Australian, South Australian and New South Wales governments also signed the statement of intent and other state and territory governments have made various commitments to improving Indigenous health.

Alongside the government initiatives, the Close the Gap campaign has continued as a non-government umbrella organisation, with some 80 peak bodies and organisations now involved. It holds meetings on a quarterly basis and produces an annual "shadow" report, to coincide with the report produced by the government highlighting the previous year's achievements by the Closing the Gap program.

Tom also played an important role in the federal Parliament's epochal "Apology" to Australia's Indigenous peoples for past laws and practices, in particular those that had produced the "Stolen Generations" of Aboriginal children forcibly removed from their families. Acknowledgement of the Stolen Generations and the damage done to both the children who had been taken and their communities was largely a product of the *Bringing Them Home* report of the Australian Human Rights Commission (AHRC), detailing the scale and effects of forcible removal. One of the recommendations of the report, tabled in federal Parliament in 1997, was that "Australian Parliaments offer official apologies and acknowledge the responsibility of their predecessors for the laws, policies, and practices of forcible removal". Between 1997 and 2001, each Australian state and territory government accepted that recommendation and apologised in Parliament to the Stolen Generations. However, while the federal government passed a motion of reconciliation in Parliament in August 1999, which expressed "deep and sincere regret", it refused to make a formal national apology.

Demand for an apology, from both the Indigenous community and the general public, nevertheless continued to build. Following the victory of the Labor Party in the federal election of November 2007, the new prime minister, Kevin Rudd, announced that an official apology would be made, the wording of which would be decided in consultation with Indigenous leaders. Tom Calma was involved in the consultative process with Stolen Generations' representative bodies, such as the National Sorry Day Committee and the Stolen Generations Alliance, who asked him to make the formal response in Parliament to the Apology, delivered on 13 February 2008. Tom did so, not simply as an advocate for his people, but as someone whose own family had been affected by the policy of forcible removal.

Other initiatives in his role as Social Justice Commissioner which Tom sees as important include the promotion of the concept of Justice Reinvestment (which he advocated in his 2009 Social Justice Report) and the establishment of the National Congress of Australia's First Peoples. Justice Reinvestment involves a proactive approach to crime prevention, seeing money more productively spent in overcoming

[12]The 2030 date was subsequently changed to 2031 to coincide with the scheduled census.

the conditions that generate crime, such as lack of education, unemployment and substance abuse, than in the costs associated with dealing with crime once it has occurred, such as the provision of prisons. Well established in a number of American states, it is attracting government interest in Australia, with an active community organisation promoting it in New South Wales.[13]

Prior to Tom's tenure at AHRC, the federal government had established the Aboriginal and Torres Strait Islander Commission (ATSIC) as a national representative body. Consistent with the philosophy of Indigenous self-determination, ATSIC both provided advice to government on policies that affected Indigenous peoples and delivered various government services. Amidst a good deal of controversy, ATSIC was decommissioned in 2004. Tom voiced his concerns over the lack of a national representative body in his 2006 Commissioner's Report, but was unable to advance representation and advocacy in 2007 due to the distraction of the Northern Territory Intervention. He released an issues paper titled "Building a Sustainable National Indigenous Representative Body—Issues for Consideration" on 12 July 2008. In December 2008 he was engaged by the federal government to facilitate consultations to develop options for such a body. Drawing on the results of an extensive process of consultation, a steering committee chaired by Tom produced the *Our Future in Our Hands* report.[14] On the basis of this report, the National Congress of Australia's First Peoples—like ATSIC, a democratically structured body representing all Indigenous peoples but, unlike ATSIC, a company limited by guarantee, operating independently of the government—was established in 2011.[15]

In the light of his commitments to a human rights approach to the social problems faced by Indigenous communities and peoples, and to an empowerment development approach in working with them to deal with the challenges, it is not surprising that in his dual roles as Social Justice Commissioner and Race Discrimination Commissioner Tom was highly critical of what has become known as the "NT Intervention".[16] The immediate catalyst for the Intervention was the release in June 2007 of the Report of the Northern Territory Board of Inquiry into the Protection of Aboriginal Children from Sexual Abuse, titled *Ampe Akelyernemane Meke Mekarle: 'Little Children are Sacred'*, detailing severe problems of child abuse and family violence in a number of Aboriginal communities. Within a week of the release of the report, the federal government announced a suite of measures that aimed to address these problems, subsequently enshrining the measures in legislation that drew on the "race powers" of the Australian Constitution and at the same time suspended the application of the Racial Discrimination Act where it conflicted with the measures. These included

---

[13]Information about Just Reinvest NSW is at http://justicereinvestmentnow.net.au/.

[14]https://www.humanrights.gov.au/publications/our-future-our-hands-2009.

[15]See http://nationalcongress.com.au/.

[16]See http://www.humanrights.gov.au/publications/social-justice-report-2007-chapter-3-northern-territory-emergency-response-intervention.

restrictions on the availability of alcohol on Aboriginal land; "income management" (also known as "welfare quarantining"), where a percentage of the welfare payments of recipients who are deemed to belong to such categories as "Disengaged Youth", "Long-term Welfare Recipients" or "Vulnerable Welfare Payment Recipients" are set aside to be spent only on "priority goods and services" (items such as food, housing, clothing, education and health care) and acquiring townships prescribed by the Australian government through five-year leases including payment of just terms of compensation. In short, the "Intervention" constituted a massive paternalistic imposition on Indigenous communities by the federal government, an imposition that it would not have been able to make on any other group. It suspended human rights protections to Northern Territory Indigenous peoples.

While supporting the ends of the Intervention to the extent they were the protection of such fundamental human rights as the right to bodily integrity and security, Tom was highly critical of the means used to achieve those ends, on both pragmatic and principled grounds. Condemning the Intervention for what he saw as a top-down approach that failed to engage with the communities it was supposed to be assisting, Tom wrote in his Social Justice Report of 2007:

> The most significant problem with the new arrangements … is the lack of capacity for engagement and participation of Indigenous peoples. This manifests as a lack of connection between the local and regional level, up to the state and national level; and as a disconnect between the making of policy and its implementation…
>
> Indigenous peoples are treated as problems to be solved, not as partners and active participants in creating a positive life vision for the generations of Indigenous peoples still to come.
>
> The greatest irony of this is that it fosters a passive system of policy development and service delivery while at the same time criticising Indigenous peoples for being passive recipients of government services!
>
> As the timeline for the introduction of the legislation vividly demonstrates, the government was unwilling to enter into any dialogue, let alone negotiations, with Indigenous communities or the broader community about the methods to be adopted. The circumscribed process for debate and scrutiny also meant there was limited scrutiny prior to the introduction of the legislation … it appears inconceivable that a program to address issues as fundamental as family violence and child abuse should be the cause of community division. Such a process should have built partnerships across society and solidified a joint determination to address the scourge of family violence and child abuse in Indigenous communities.
>
> Instead, the approach adopted has created or exacerbated division and mistrust between the federal government, the Northern Territory government, Indigenous communities and numerous community organisations.
>
> The introduction of the NT intervention has, as a result, been highly controversial.
>
> The responsibility for creating such division lies with those who led the process. The inability to develop a national consensus and partnership for addressing violence and abuse should be seen as one of the main legacies, and a significant failure, of the now former Minister for Indigenous Affairs.

Tom left the AHRC in 2010, when he also decided not to return to the Public Service, but he has continued to lead an active and highly productive public life. He has held or holds posts such as the Chair of the Commonwealth Government's Aboriginal and Torres Strait Islander Suicide Prevention Advisory Group and member of their Aboriginal and Torres Strait Islander Mental Health Advisory Group, Co-Chair of the Aboriginal and Torres Strait Islander Mental Health and Suicide Prevention Advisory Group, an Ambassador with Suicide Prevention Australia, an Adjunct Associate Professor at the National Centre for Indigenous Studies at ANU, the inaugural National Coordinator for Tackling Indigenous Smoking (Commonwealth Department of Health and Ageing), Co-Chair of Reconciliation Australia, Co-Chair of the Indigenous Community Volunteers network, member of the Australian Social Inclusion Board, National Patron of the Poche Centres for Indigenous Health, Chair of the Cooperative Research Centre for Remote Economic Participation and Ninti One Ltd., a member of the Law Advisory Council of the University of New South Wales and is a chair or member of numerous other national boards, committees and campaigns. Recently Tom was appointed as one of two external members of the Commonwealth Secretaries Equality and Diversity Council.[17]

Tom estimates that he makes one major speech or presentation a week, focusing on Indigenous health, Indigenous mental health, Indigenous empowerment, economic development and reconciliation.[18]

In one way or another, virtually all Tom's efforts continue the work he did at the AHRC to raise awareness of the place of Indigenous peoples in Australian society, and the problems they face—and to empower them to address them.

As cited at the beginning of this chapter, over the past few years Tom has received official recognition for his achievements and contribution to Australian society, receiving honorary doctorates, being made an Officer of the Order of Australia (AO), being named the ACT Australian of the Year in 2013, and in 2014 appointed Chancellor of the University of Canberra, the first Indigenous person to become chancellor of an Australian university.

Tom readily acknowledges that this personal recognition could only be achieved because he has the support of his wife, Heather, and his three children, who have all followed him into professions that serve others. He also credits his successes to the foundation that was laid by his parents and extended family and the community development and social work studies he undertook, along with many Aboriginal and Torres Strait Islander people from across the nation.

[17]See https://www.dpmc.gov.au/office-women/secretaries-equality-and-diversity-council.

[18]A full list of Tom Calma's publications and presentations is available at http://ncis.anu.edu.au/_lib/doc/publications_Tom.pdf.

Analysis of Qualities/Character

Commitment

For most of his working life Tom has not been employed as a social worker in terms of designations of his positions. Nevertheless, his training as a social worker has been foundational to his way of thinking and practice, and much of his work, particularly since taking up his roles with the AHRC, can be seen as reflecting the commitment which led him into social work in the first place, and drawing on the techniques and skills that he learnt, or further developed, there. His approach to societal change through free, prior and informed consent, empowerment and people-centred development has pervaded his work ethos and practice. In the biographic interview, Tom often identified with social work training and community development knowledge, and he used it in a range of positions he served in with engagement and commitment.

Practical Wisdom

Tom has had a conspicuously successful and productive working life. Moreover, his working life has developed naturally from his personal experience and values (relationship with Aboriginal land and people). He has consistently exhibited practical wisdom in his work, finding ways to achieve the goals that he has set, in particular by building coalitions of like-minded individuals and organisations, and setting realistic and achievable goals to move towards desirable outcomes.

Tom himself has developed the skills he needed to exercise practical wisdom in the area in which he wanted to be effective—empowerment of disadvantaged communities—from an early age. In the first instance this was, of course, a matter of natural inclination, guidance by others, especially his parents, and opportunities that he availed himself of to provide assistance and exercise leadership. As he became older, however, he actively sought out ways of developing the explicit knowledge and technical skills he needed. He did this firstly by developing his skills in administration and community sector engagement then gaining an education in social work and community development. He relates, for example, that when his children were small he became a member of their primary school council, and eventually its chair, an experience which provided him with valuable understanding of governance and administration and the relationship between them—understanding which served him well in future work.

Big-Picture Person

From the very beginning, Tom was a big-picture person. Thinking and planning big is an important quality that only a small number of people cultivate. Tom said: *But I very clearly was a big-picture person and a lot of the work that we did was big picture.*

He acknowledges the importance of work with individuals, but he thinks one could not do a lot with such an approach. To him societal circumstances have to be changed to change individual circumstances: *Working with individual families over a long time you could make a change, but the real big change came when there was an attitudinal change and people were able to go through school and see education as a worthy practice.*

A lot of policies, planning and programs Tom was involved in were of macro practice nature at the national level.

Quest for Creating Opportunities

Thinking big and creating opportunities go together. In the biographic narration, Tom often referred to creating opportunities. In several capacities in public service, he has tried to create opportunities for Aboriginal people and communities, and others alike. Tom confirms how creating opportunities helps:

> I know it works and I know it works for Aboriginal people that when given the opportunity in a really genuine way, in a way that's supportive and … yeah, I suppose, and encouraging, then Aboriginal people will succeed, and we've seen that over and over again. Where it breaks down and it fails is when somebody tries to dictate about what happens or they try and apply a policy that's the one size fits all, irrespective of your sort of background or experience or whatever, or they don't look at the determinants of why a person is in their predicament, where they're starting from, and it's all about government, and this is the worst thing about governments is that they want to achieve things within a very short timeframe and particularly within a political cycle, they want to get some big gains and rewards so they can hang their cap on, and they don't realise how destabilising that is and how inefficient that is.

At Right Place, at Right Time with Right People

Tom's ability to make personal connections with a very broad range of people has been a great assistance to him in his career and professional activities. No doubt this reflects, at least to some extent, Tom's personable nature. He relates that when as a young man he joined the public service in Darwin as a base-grade clerk, through his father he was introduced to the senior manager of the department he worked in, George Redman, the State Director. The two men discovered that they shared a love of fishing. Soon Tom was showing Redman how to fish for barramundi in creeks, while Redman taught him how to game fish. These fishing trips provided time for extended discussions about how things were done in the public service, from which Tom learned much. In a meeting, he sat next to the Department Secretary, who at the end of the meeting offered him a position in Canberra. *So it's been fortunate I've been in the right place at the right time.*

But again, Tom developed his capacity to get on with others through his social work education and experience. So, he credits his ability to liaise effectively with representatives of different elements of the higher education and vocational training sectors in India to the skills and approaches he learned in his group work and community training and practice: *skills that I learnt in community development in social work that were able to assist me in starting to communicate and develop relationships with people in India.*

Respect for Autonomy, Self-control/Determination and Empowerment

While social work places a good deal of emphasis on the importance of respect for autonomy, social workers, like many professionals, are often faced with situations where they desire to improve the situation of clients who resist help, or are unable to persist with the course of action that will assist them. In such situations paternalism—acting to help another, despite or irrespective of that person's own wishes—is a standing temptation. Tom's practice and philosophy consistently stress respect for autonomy and self-determination as basic precepts of ethical and effective practice. This essentially entails power of listening and empowering others to take control of their life situation or knowing where and how to access support:

> all of this is founded around making people the centre of the issue that needs to be resolved and to empower people to take control of their own lives …
>
> they can be the solution brokers and be party to addressing the issues that confront their life as distinct from trying to change a person's life in a more aggressive way.
>
> To be able to give people enough information to make informed decisions [is a] key tenet of what we learnt in social work and being able to push that and instil that agenda which I think is most important.

Tom also devotes time to educating policy makers and influencers about the paradigms of social and cultural determinants and how they impact on the well-being of individuals and groups. He suggests we stop blaming people and begin listening to them:

> there's a long history of failed experiments by government that are blamed on the people, and that sort of rhetoric's got to stop and we've got to get down to some meaningful engagement.

In terms of listening, Tom did not find anyone being real champions of Indigenous Affairs among politicians. He said:

> Most of them listen to the Party or do their own thing…
>
> all of them, none of them are really stand-outs as being real champions, in my view, because they're too much influenced by their own interests and the interests of the Party, which becomes a political interest rather than a people interest. Too few are interested in applied research findings and those who are interested, are backbenchers or from the minor Parties …
>
> if we were able to maintain a determinants approach and an empowerment development approach that we took with the Close the Gap campaign, then I'm sure that Aboriginal Affairs would be a different place than what it is now.

Tom emphasised that understanding, empathy and power of discussion and listening are really important. He suggests understanding causes and developing broader approaches to changing it by engaging, empowering and encouraging people to join, *without trying to dictate to people about how to run their lives*. Tom believes not following such an approach results in apathy:

> I very much believe that we shouldn't be just creating new initiatives for the sake of new initiatives but work out what's working and building on that and if there's something that's not working then work out why it's not working and work around that issue rather than to just say alright, forget that and we'll go on to something else because a bureaucrat or politician might have a whiz bang idea but by the time it gets down to the community level and the community understanding, it could take years and many different iterations in the process and that just creates a sort of despondency with people and that same despondency is recognised or is portrayed by government as a lack of listening and apathy. And it is apathy but it's just apathy that's been developed because of the way policies change.

Courage

Although Tom is clearly a highly diplomatic person, who prefers to operate by gaining consensus and building alliances rather than by confrontation, he has shown courage in his willingness to speak forthrightly to powerbrokers and politicians when he judges it necessary, as demonstrated in his comments about the Intervention quoted above. Tom talked about courage as follows:

> they need to have the fortitude to be able to let things run their course, to let Aboriginal and Torres Strait Islander people make mistakes and let us address those mistakes instead of Government trying to orchestrate that all the time …
>
> I just had to knuckle down and have faith in myself and just keep on going.

Diplomacy and Strategic Thinking and Planning

Tom uniquely combines the qualities of diplomacy and strategic thinking and planning. Within a bureaucratic context, working around contested issues—such as human rights, Aboriginal land rights, amendment to laws, reconciliation, Closing the Gap agenda, the national Apology to Aboriginal people and communities, mobilising people and organisations, and initiating change—requires, beyond commitment, sophisticated diplomacy and strategic planning and thinking. In a range of positions where Tom has worked, from vocational officer to human rights commissioner, he has clearly demonstrated these qualities.

Achievement Orientation

The analysis of biographic interview data clearly showed that Tom is an achievement and success oriented person and professional, as he often focused on career achievements and successes: establishing vocational training programs, starting new educational courses with good enrolments, building an agents' association in India and alumni network in Vietnam,[19] outcomes of the Close the Gap movement, bringing the peak bodies together, responding to the national Apology, attaining the ranks of Social Justice and Race Discrimination commissioners and chancellor. In regard to media coverage, Tom states: *journalists sensationalise, they focus on a deficit model instead of looking at achievements and outcomes, which is a real shame*.

As discussed below, Tom's achievement drive does not suggest that he did not learn from his failures and all experiences, but his focus on achievements demonstrates what drives the person to accomplish what he has accomplished in his life. Tom also believes strongly in mentoring and developing other interested parties and he selflessly lends his time to such endeavours.

Continuous Learning

Continuous learning is crucial for one's own and others' growth and development. Tom's life story shows how he practised learning from every new exposure and experience. As stated above, he learned from his interaction with public servants and similar experiences, both nationally and internationally: *So there was a lot of merit in that and so I got to understand all of those sorts of processes and got to meet a lot of politicians and their staff and a lot of senior bureaucrats*.

---

[19]See point 2 at this link—http://vgac.net/about-us/ It was a defunct body and Tom Calma co-led its resurrection.

In the context of Aboriginal communities, Tom believes that both learning and unlearning are necessary:

> I think in (pause) – we've got to learn in some areas how to develop relationships, how to experience life without alcohol or tobacco, we've got to unlearn that nexus that's been developed between tobacco and lifestyle remembering that up until the late 1960s early 1970s many Aboriginal people in remote Australia were paid rations including tobacco, so there's been a big culture of smoking and we've got to unlearn that culture and relearn what a healthy lifestyle is about. I think we've got to (pause) learn about how do we address lateral violence and that's basically talking about each other amongst our own people, talking in a derogatory manner. We've got to learn to respect each other a lot more.

Working Together/Collective Work and Building Teams and Movements

Tom has clearly demonstrated the qualities of team building and working together and creating movements. This was quite obvious in the work he did overseas as a counsellor. Back home, he mobilised peak bodies to work together on the Close the Gap agenda, worked along with national peak bodies to respond to the national Apology, just to name a few. To Tom, the Close the Gap campaign has become a people movement, with a national Close the Gap Day. The following shows the collective work approach of Tom:

> collectively we need to try and share with each other and with those who are in positions of influence that there are different ways to do things and I'm sure that this will work …
>
> bringing individuals together and having a shared and collective understanding to move away from an adversarial role with governments and politicians to one of having a very diplomatic approach to the way we do things and making sure that it's respectful.
>
> Well the key thing when taking on a controversial issue is to do it as a group. As an individual you can very easily be picked off. As a group, you know of collective minds, you can assert and influence a lot more.

Initiating New Projects/Change and Leading

Throughout his career, Tom has initiated or was offered opportunities to initiate new projects and lead them. At the beginning of his career he headed the courses and curriculum development, directed employment skill development and training programs. In his overseas assignments he facilitated the development of an agents' association with a code of conduct, established new offices in many countries and helped establish the Vietnam Graduates from Australia Club. He worked diligently for the Close the Gap agenda and authored social justice reports that looked at human rights violations and argued for making necessary changes. He is also a great supporter of the philosophy of justice reinvestment. Many people have ideas, but the difference with Tom is that he fructifies by leading them.

Activism with Diplomacy

In most of his career Tom was in the public service, where any kind of activism is difficult to achieve by being an insider. But activism does not always mean street marches; it can also be about challenging conventional thinking, identifying and offering solutions to wicked problems and it can also be about educating and informing people about culturally acceptable practices and behaviours. By looking at his work in various positions and his stand on certain issues, we think Tom has achieved significant activism and diplomacy in his practice. Some of his thoughts of activism may be inferred from the following:

> Australia as a colonial white society has been a significant contributor to many of the problems experienced by Aboriginal and Torres Strait Islander peoples. To meaningfully address many issues of the past we must move beyond the national Apology and address things like reconciliation, a treaty and recognition in the Constitution of the First Peoples.

Tom has argued well and/or supported a case of amending relevant provisions of the Australian Constitution (for example, Section 25, 51.26, 116a, 127a) that discriminate and do not recognise Aboriginal people. Tom's activism may also be seen in relation to health issues (Closing the Gap, smoking, alcohol and drugs, suicide, mental health, and social and emotional wellbeing) in Aboriginal communities. Tom questions the following and has been working for that important cause:

> You know, if we have a major disaster in Australia in any community, governments generally do not go into the community and start restructuring that community without first engaging with the people and hearing what the people want to do and how they want to go about doing it. The moment it comes to Aboriginal land the governments believe they have a right to go and dictate to Aboriginal people. Why should we be treated differently to other citizens of Australia? And this sort of happens, and it's because of the mindset of politicians and the community who can't see the difference; they always see Aboriginal people as a different class of citizen in Australia. I know that's a big statement, but when practices happen like that, then that's the only explanation or conclusion one can draw. My goal is to raise awareness about this, to expose this, to try and make sure that governments do take a lot more consideration of our people. I, like many of my people, say, "Do things with us and not to us".

Focus and Consistency

Drawing on his experience, Tom insisted that it is important to remain focused and consistent. He believes that too often *there is no sound policy reason for change;*

it's ideology or it's of personal interest. Lack of consistent policy is the main problem. Referring to many reports (for example, *A Strategic Review of Indigenous Expenditure*, Andrew Forrest Review, COAG trials and more recently the Indigenous Advancement Strategy reforms), Tom said:

> governments have failed in Indigenous Affairs because they haven't had a consistent approach that has been stop-start, and that it's been imposed from the centre and from Canberra. And you know, and we all know, that in the policy arena, many bureaucrats know that, but politicians don't get it, and it's not Indigenous people saying it; these are mainstream bodies that are saying the same thing and so it then becomes only ideology that's driving the way Indigenous public policy has been done.

However, in his practice, Tom said, *I try to practise being consistent and applying those same principles in everyday life wherever you can.*

If we do not remain focused and consistent, we go backwards. In Tom's words:

> and that's why it's so critical that we have the Close the Gap campaign and that governments sign up and stay very focused in trying to have a long-term strategy, a generational approach and stay very focused and committed, and that commitment includes no big changes in policy direction, no stop-start in funding, no taking U-turns and bloody left turns and right turns in policy, because all that does, every time that happens we see a despondency within the community and a lack of faith in bureaucracy and government, and we go backwards.

Voluntary and Philanthropic Work

Tom's life story shows his deep interest in voluntary and philanthropic work: *I wanted to do a lot more philanthropic work and other work back in the community. And so that [retirement in 2010] would give me an opportunity to do that.*

He terms his retirement as a *pseudo retirement* as since retirement he has been engaged in both paid and philanthropic work, which he enjoys. Tom leads and serves on numerous committees and missions, and organisations. Simply, the space does not allow listing them here, but a Wikipedia search will reveal them.[20]

Humility

Tom seems to have internalised the quality of humility from his father, who well demonstrated people management skills, humanity and humility to his colleagues. In regard to supporting the aspirations of a fledgling Aboriginal band, Tom humbly admits the following:

---

[20]See https://en.wikipedia.org/wiki/Tom_Calma.

> if they only relied on my initial assessment as a delegate they wouldn't have cut their first tape, I wouldn't approve it, but I was convinced in the end and I did approve it. If I hadn't had my mind changed where would Yothu Yindi be now? But it just shows that you sometimes don't make the best decision, but you should always have an open mind and be willing to eat humble pie.

About his Human Rights Commission work, Tom said:

> I'm not the font of all knowledge, but in talking with people and working through issues with people, we come up with solutions. So that's the collective nature of what we do. That's epitomised in the way that the Human Rights Commission works or worked …
>
> the work around suicide which wasn't just me, it was a whole lot of us and I led it …
>
> a true leader is someone who has ideas, is willing to listen to other people's ideas and in arriving at a position, all parties walk together to progress the initiative.

Despite uncommon accomplishments, Tom admitted his limitations and gave due credit to others, which shows some aspects of his humility.

Conclusion

Tom Calma's biography presents a compelling story of his development from a relatively disadvantaged context and insights from his life experiences of relative poverty, health issues, discrimination, timely association and opportunities. Remaining humble, he has shown extraordinary leadership in Australian public life and demonstrated practical wisdom emanating from a combination of Aboriginal culture and social work knowledge and skills, and their application.

Chapter 5
Respect and Integrity—John Gavaghan

A.W. (Bill) Anscombe and Emma Rush

Positively and universally respected by those who know of his work, John Gavaghan is known for his commitment to clients, unfailing fairness, warmth and good humour, optimism and hope, and an ability to courageously tackle difficult and entrenched issues while operating reflectively and in the interests of others. He has been described as a man who is able to integrate the compassion of the heart with the intellect of the head.

John has worked for the majority of his life in the area of child protection in two New South Wales government departments (although one has had numerous name changes). Prior to retirement in 2010, John held the position of Director of Child and Family Services, which included areas of significant disadvantage in south-west Sydney and some of the most entrenched urban areas of poverty and disadvantage. A measure of the man is that since his retirement at age 60, he has repeatedly been asked back into child protection to manage some of the most difficult rural and remote offices of the state. In a long, stable and supportive marriage, John and his wife have two adult children.

Family Background

John is one of six children who grew up sharing their family home with multiple foster-care children. Born in 1950, John's early life was happy and full of the events and activities of children growing up in a new outer suburb of Sydney, with

A.W. (Bill) Anscombe (✉) · E. Rush
Charles Sturt University, Wagga Wagga, Australia
e-mail: BAnscombe@csu.edu.au

E. Rush
e-mail: erush@csu.edu.au

M. Pawar et al. (eds.), *Empowering Social Workers*,
DOI 10.1007/978-981-10-3809-9_5

opportunities for unstructured play in a climate of trust and the opportunity for childhood risk taking. He says:

> I suppose some of the early interest in doing what I'm doing now was stimulated by the fact that my mother was a carer and had foster kids in the family … when I was about six or seven I think, we had a young bloke join our family and he was with us for about three or four years until the time I was about ten. I'd had a fairly close relationship to this young boy… he was a year or two younger I think … and was a part of our family. He eventually went back to his family because there was some work done at that time to re-establish him back in his family of origin.
>
> So it was from those early days that I was probably interested in the fact that not all families are the same. Our family was certainly different—although we were middle class—not well to do—in fact, fairly impoverished. There was no sewerage or anything like that and so it was a fairly basic sort of existence. So it was from those early days I think when I look back there was some interest even at that point about the fact that people come from different environments.
>
> But I remember C … very well. I don't think my mother was quite clear about how she was going to break the news to me that he was going to be leaving the family. So I was really distressed around the time when he actually left the family and went back to his family.

Almost 50 years later, John describes the following:

> We were celebrating Children's Week … the Minister was invited to this celebration where the Playback Theatre asked for participation from the audience about people who wanted to recall some memory of childhood. I remembered this time when C … and I were together and he was about to return to his family, and it was an incredibly distressing time for me. I felt at that stage, the same sorts of emotions that I felt 50 years earlier when this boy left; it was an unbelievably powerful experience that the players were representing because they captured exactly the sorts of feelings that I had about this boy, and he'd gone and I didn't know where he'd gone to. And it was always in the back of my mind that these sorts of things were somehow or other to do with me, and I'd wondered why it was that this boy had gone. What had I done? And they were able to capture this moment just exquisitely to the point where I literally burst out crying in the middle of this Playback presentation, and in the audience of 100 or so… there was the Minister sitting in the front row watching one of her staff members blubbering away about how he'd been affected by the separation of this ten-year-old boy and her ten-year-old staff member at the time.
>
> This was a really significant event for me because it showed her that the manager that she'd actually had appointed to a position in charge of several other staff at that stage was able to be so affected by the separation of this young boy from himself as a manager that 50 years later it was still impacting upon him. And I thought I was very fortunate in lots of ways that she could see me being so distressed and upset by that episode, and it got her, I think, to realise that separation is a major issue that children face whenever they move from one family to another, which is the reason why I think I've got so much interest in making sure that everything is done to maintain a family intact before children are removed from that family and placed in some other environment that they're not familiar with.
>
> And it was a quite a fascinating review and reflection about how something as straightforward and simple as that could have such an impact so many years down the track, an impact for me because it was something which provided me with an invaluable experience about how much attachment affects subsequent relationship…

> And even after that episode I was in touch with a couple of the Playback Theatre members … and said how appreciative I was that they'd been able to capture my experience as a ten year old so exactly. It was a brilliant episode … I was literally able to release some of those sorts of feelings of separation that I had which I obviously hadn't released before.

The Influence of Schooling

John attended nearby Riverview College, to which he won a scholarship. He describes Riverview as a fantastic school that provided an incredibly broad, rounded education. There were children and young people at Riverview who were exceptionally well to do (unlike John's family) and others from a range of different backgrounds. This further stimulated an interest in the fact that people are different and that they can constructively work together in a different environment. He considers that if the environment that fosters that difference is able to join people together, what they are separately able to bring, usually benefits all of the people. It stimulated his interest in working with difference—an interest in different cultures, different languages, different family orientations and different orientations generally. He recognised that when he sees a marginalised group that needs to be included, there are some qualities in him that force him to think about what else could be happening in the environment that might lead to a different outcome for people. He describes this as a

> sort of a guiding principle so that the sorts of things that I do as a professional would be very much predicated on what the benefit is to this person in being in this situation at this time. Is there something which they would want to do, or might want to do, that could contribute to getting to a different place that's going to be more satisfactory for them than being exactly where they are at the moment? This is not to suggest that being where they are at the moment is not good enough, but it is to suggest that if there's a desire on their part to change the circumstances that they're in, then they in fact end up making and are responsible for and controlling the destiny of that making. It was that which really guided me to become involved in social work when I was a more mature adolescent.

Riverview was a school devoted to sporting prowess, which John did not have (although he described himself as the best full-back that the eighth division rugby team ever had!). Formal schooling and opportunities were matched by informal events that profoundly affected him. In one such event an exceptionally gifted student was giving an oration. The topic was the importance of truth and he spoke about the moment in Shakespeare's *Hamlet* when Laertes is asking Polonius what it is that he should take with him in his travels to a far distant place. Polonius said to Laertes, "This above all—to thine own self be true, and it must follow, as the night the day, thou canst not then be false to any man." John thought this was what captured Riverview: it was about the way in which people are truthful to one another in their day-to-day deliberations. John described it as moving and so powerful.

University

Leaving school, social work was an interest that was not formulated well and, in hindsight, John considered that his reasons for getting into social work were not profound, with much more interest in the social aspect of university. The costs associated with going through university at that time (1968) were fairly extensive and at the end of his first year his father said, "Look, you're going to have to make a decision about either getting a scholarship or getting a job, because I can't afford to keep you at university anymore". The public service was offering generous cadetships, so John applied for one and was successful with entry to the (then) Department of Child Welfare and Social Welfare. He effectively had a three-year scholarship in a four-year degree. The scholarship offered a living allowance, a book allowance, the costs of living day to day, a wage over the vacations between terms, working with the Department, and a guarantee of a job after graduating. It was an incentive to stay at university. A condition of the scholarship was to be prepared to be employed by the Department for four years.

Employment

John found the work fascinating, as it involved working with families, working with difference, and with people whose lives had been fractured in one sense or another. Children in some family environments needed something different from that to which they have been exposed. He was challenged by working with some of the families where things had gone dramatically wrong and kids were being terribly injured, including cigarette burns on arms and feet, deliberately inflicted broken bones and fractures and punches and bruises. He recognised that sometimes parents had absolutely no idea about how to discipline or deal with the sorts of challenges that parenthood provided, with the consequence that they lashed out whenever things got too much, to the detriment of the children. These experiences connected him to the profession.

After a year of personal travel (which he saw as almost a prescribed requirement for new graduates), he returned to Community Services, where he stayed for five years. He then moved to the Department of Health in the inner-city area of Sydney, where the job was working with people who were marginalised and isolated through homelessness or drug dependence. This stimulated an interest in the range of social services available to individuals and families. After two years, John moved within the Department of Health to the position of Co-ordinator of Regional Child Abuse Programs. The approach involved disciplines working together for child protection and child abuse prevention. In the late 1970s, child protection was largely the province of medical staff, doctors and paediatric staff who dealt with children when they entered the health system because of injuries. The whole area of abuse in families was still in its infancy, though there'd been quite a few years of experience in the USA, through Henry Kempe's work. Some of that work was what John was particularly interested in when still with the Department of Child Welfare and Social Welfare, before moving to Health. The experience in that early part of his career allowed him to connect with health professionals who were, at that point, starting to see the relevance of the work that Kempe was doing.

The Department of Child Welfare and Social Welfare at that stage emphasised neglect, where the legislative provisions of the Child Welfare Act included concepts like "exposed to moral danger" and "family dysfunction", but there was rarely a focus on inflicted injury. John says:

> Starting my profession at the time when that change and that impetus was only starting to gather pace was a really fascinating time. And Health's involvement in its paediatric services together with the sort of legislative constraints that Community Services was able to muster was an interesting meeting place, because it hadn't happened before, and when it did happen it was quite demonstrable that you could do things with families where there was the use of some statutory power to change the dynamics of what was happening in a family. That became a real focus for me for many, many years, and probably still is. It stimulated an interest in working in Health, but it also stimulated an interest in doing some longer-term work back in Community Services, which I eventually came back into.
>
> But while I was in Health I actually built up quite a solid network of people who were able to offer services that could be consumed by families—services like drug and alcohol services, infant health, early infancy education, and all of the sorts of things that families need if they're going to provide the sort of structure that's necessary for kids to survive and grow and develop. And they became pretty much a going concern that I had about what would be really useful for families to have if they were interested in their children getting the best out of the environment within that family. So when I came back into Family and Community Services ... I had the inkling of what it was like to work in an environment where people worked together, where disciplines worked together, where teams worked together, and where professions worked together.
>
> I started to look at some of the sorts of changes that you could practically get out of those disciplines providing a service together, rather than out of those individual professions providing another service separately... it actually stimulated people to think about, "What don't I know that somebody else does, and how might that information be of use to a family which needs the knowledge that one person's got, together with the knowledge that another person's got?" Even if they're not within the same person, and I suppose that's been a sort of a guiding principle as well; you don't need to know everything, but you do need to know that other people have got knowledge that you mightn't have. And it's that ability to recognise the knowledge that you don't have and the capacity that somebody else has to actually provide something that a family might need which can benefit both yourself and the other professional, and more particularly the family who requires what you both are able to marshal. Those sorts of dynamics really quite stimulated me to work back in Community Services, to see whether we could use that earlier experience of people working together to provide for families what they might not have been able to get by people working separately.

After ten years in Health, John moved into the Family Crisis Service of what was then the Department of Family and Community Services. This was an after-business-hours service that frequently responded to crises occurring after normal business hours. The idea of working with families in crisis was a particular interest, because of an early experience in drawing together the range of skills that different disciplines could bring to provide useful services to families. The service was one point where the difficulties that a family was experiencing could be identified, and then the range of services that were available could be marshalled for that family to be able to provide somewhat different parenting of their children. When that was not possible, then the legislative processes had to be embarked upon, and then children and families were separated.

That separation became a real interest for John too, because whatever you think about how families were providing for their children, children were familiar with their environment and there was going to be a loss when they were extracted from that environment and had to endure something else. That notion of loss and grief around change was something that John found stimulating and perplexing, because he could see that it was necessary for children to be removed from environments that were volatile and placed them at significant risk, but he could also see that they experienced some damage as a result of being removed from the environments where they had significant connections and placed into other environments where they didn't have those connections. That was particularly the case with Indigenous children who, at that stage, were extracted without really any form of proper assessment being undertaken as to what they were being extracted from, and without any proper assessment of what they were being provided with once they were placed elsewhere.

John worked for the remainder of his career within Community Services, where he managed a range of offices in metropolitan Sydney and finally had responsibility for them as Director of Child and Family Services for Metropolitan South-West. Since retirement he has managed rural and remote locations as the manager of Client Services.

Analysis of Qualities/Character

At the heart of John's social work and personal life is a commitment to diversity, a valuing of human dignity and the importance of reflective practice, as can be gleaned from the narratives that he recounts in relation to his childhood, education and work history. Other salient features include equity of access and entitlement; the importance of respect, listening, values and the need for reflective practice; and relationships built on mutual respect, trust and vulnerability.

Equity of access and entitlement is a key consideration. In discussing rural and remote locations John commented on the level of inconsistency in the provision of services and how different service provision can disadvantage people.

> In Bourke, or in Goodooga or in any of the other more outlying parts of the state, inconsistency impacted upon what might happen in a family. In one area for instance, it might well have been possible for the family to have remained intact, and yet in exactly the same sorts of dynamics in the other area it could lead to the whole lot being fractured. And those sorts of things just did not make sense to me. So I was really interested in trying to get an approach which was much more consistent across the agencies—how they would need

to marshal the availability of their services so that more or less the same sorts of services were available to communities no matter where they existed.

It was that impetus for consistency, the nub of which was that families are entitled to, and children are entitled to, support which provides them with an opportunity to do something different about how the parenting practices in a family could unfold for the children. And that seemed to me to be a really critical issue, that it didn't make any difference where you lived—you were entitled to have people listen to you and you were entitled to have people offer you the sorts of services that you didn't have access to that allowed you to do what the children in that family required and needed if they were going to be able to grow to their full potential.

Other important qualities are the importance of respect, listening, values and the need for reflective practice. John says:

A lot of the work that I'm doing now is again about how you actually demonstrate respect; how do you demonstrate the value that you want to show when you're operating with integrity; how do you actually demonstrate that you are somebody who is fair and open; and how do you demonstrate trust? Those sorts of things are pretty critical to me. When Carmel Niland came to be the Director General at Community Services… she took an interesting approach and one of the first things she did was to try and get the agency to identify all of the values that it saw as being absolutely fundamental to the operation of a human service entity. And she worked with a fairly significant group of the senior staff, and also the middle managers and the case workers, and looked to identify what were the five key critical things that the agency espoused as its values and the things which it held so dear that they were virtually inviolable … she did actually get those values identified. And the people who she was working with had to know what they were, and they had to actually demonstrate them and be part of those values. And if they couldn't, then they really weren't part of that organisation.

I thought that was a fantastically successful move, and probably successful for me because it actually did seem like they were the sorts of things that allowed for people to form relationships and build change opportunities for families so that they could actually move into a different way of relating to one another which allowed for children to grow and develop. And those sorts of things were really fundamental in the way I approached my involvement in the profession.

Associated with the concepts of respect and listening is the broader concept of social work attentiveness. John made frequent reference to the importance of non-verbal cues, including facial expressions, posture and gestures. He referred to the importance of "what is not said" and the "underlying dynamics of silence". He spoke of the importance of choosing words carefully and understanding what social workers would refer to as the "meta-communication".

John recognises the importance of progressive learning, practice wisdom and reflection on practice. His comments seem to indicate that values and virtues are a framework within which reflective practice operates.

Having something [values] that you could hang onto and feel that there was some sense of reality in was a really critical feature of how I approached the whole notion of social work and the whole notion of learning how to be a practitioner. You built upon what you had; you reviewed what you actually did; you discarded things which were not going to be useful; you learnt from the things that you were reading about and consuming—to see what you could do that you hadn't done before; you got rid of the things that you could see weren't producing the things that you needed to produce; and you did and tried the elements of new theory so that you could in fact improve whatever it was that you hadn't improved before.

The importance of humility or modesty, ability to listen and the capacity to recognise his own limitations are important.

I don't know that I've been 100 per cent successful all the time; I think that'd be a bit arrogant really to say that… you think, "Well, did I really actually do as good a job on this as I thought I could have done?" And at times you're forced to admit, "No, I didn't," and I really ought to have been a little more receptive to something that I hadn't been receptive to. I should have listened more, I should have actually heard, and you can only do that when you listen properly. It makes you think, it is quite hard to listen, but unless you do it, you're never going to be able to hear properly, and you're not really ever going to relate to somebody's experience because you actually haven't demonstrated that you've understood what they're talking about. You don't have to experience the same thing but you've certainly got to hear what it's all about. And if you don't hear what it's all about there's no way in the world you're going to understand what the experience is that they've been through. So I think those sorts of things, they became fairly critical to me as I practised the profession.

The key values are highlighted as John reflects:

The DoCS values are well inculcated in my brain—the first five were fairness, openness, trust, teamwork and respect. And the two that were added [by a later Director General] were excellence and integrity. Now you can probably imagine that it would be possible to accommodate those additional two in the first five anyway, but they were separated. Integrity is pretty central. They do align with my values.

Integrity's something that you've got at your very heart from Day One onwards, and you either agree to abide by certain principles or you get out. And that's more or less what it amounts to. And if you can't abide by those sorts of principles then you really don't have an option; you've got to get out. That particular issue of integrity I think is really near and dear to me because when people make a commitment they need to stick with that commitment. And if they can't … they need to say why they can't… if you look at integrity as the ability to be fair dinkum and honest and upfront with people, which is pretty much what social work is about… then if you're able to do those things it's hard to see that somebody will denigrate whatever attempts you make to deliver something which may be of benefit to them, whatever circumstances they're in. So that's a pretty crucial notion to me. Integrity is such a fundamental part of your approach towards the way you live your life, in the way you're honest in your relationships with people and the way you respect other people, that it's a fundamental part of your existence; it's a fundamental part of my existence.

There is a real sense in which John values people rather than labels, and the implied power structures. He comments:

And how I actually regard people—I don't really see people who we're offering services to as clients as such—they're people. And there's a difference between the way the profession categorises people when they're called clients, and I suppose there's a difference between [the way] medicine categorises people when they're called patients. And there's a certain sort of distance about pushing this notion of another person away from you by calling them a client or by calling them a patient. You know, when you work in Indigenous communities, if you ever use the term "patients" or "clients" there, you'd probably get strung up because people there don't want to be seen as clients or patients, they want to be seen as people.

Conflict and judgements are an integral part of social work. John recounted a complex example that revolved around an eight-month-old Indigenous child and a legal challenge at the Supreme Court. The matter of child custody and fostering can be very complicated, with competing rights and interests.

> I was basically asked to represent the Department's view that the child should stay with the Indigenous carers who were non-kin carers. I had to brief a barrister, saying, "This is the position we have arrived at." The barrister was circumspect about taking on the case, understandably, because it was thought that this was probably an unwinnable matter. But nevertheless he accepted the case… I thought there was no way we should have allowed things to progress to this point. We should have pulled out of this case. But we didn't do that, and as a result in the Supreme Court, after a few days of hearing, when it was quite obvious that we were going to be wasting the court's time because the court would have eventually decided to place the child back in the care of the kin carers and the family of origin… I said to the barrister, "We're going to have to pull the plug on this, and I'll tell the Director General why." So I did and the Director General at least supported withdrawing the application. But on reflection I should have said early, "This is not an appropriate course to take. We're operating outside of the legislative provisions. We'll deal with the grief and loss issues that you deal with as an agency, we'll support whatever you need to do to provide ongoing support to these people who are the non-kin carers, but this child needs to be going back to where it's come from."

John believes that relationships should be built on mutual respect, trust and vulnerability. He said:

> I was in Bourke and an Indigenous colleague was welcoming the audience and giving the orientation… pointing out that Indigenous people had existed in the country for 60,000 years while some white folks had come along in the last breath and told them all how to do things differently… He was so powerful in what he was saying about the … changes that this last breath's worth of white folks' intervention had created for his community… I started crying. I thought, "Oh my God, this man is so powerful in what he's actually saying." And I was there ready to give the Sorry Day address, and did, and at the end of it we could see that we were both quite upset, and we just hugged each other and I said to him, "My tears are splashing on your shoulder," and he just held me. I thought, "Isn't that wonderful, that you can demonstrate that level of respect for one another?" And he allowed me to demonstrate it, and he did with me, and I thought, "I've formed a new relationship here." And from that time onwards we've become close colleagues… but it's relationship which has allowed the connection to develop between people in that community.
>
> And I felt enormously privileged to be able to be in his company because of the fact that he had received me in the way he had received me, and I wasn't embarrassed about letting my tears spill on his shoulder because of the impact he'd had upon me. And it was such an enormously powerful experience that I thought, "I'm really appreciative of this". I've got a genuine respect for what he wants to do for his community. And it's no more or less than he wants his community listened to, he wants his community respected, he wants his community to be able to say the things that are important to them, and he wants that listened to and respected by people who are from a different environment when they come into his country and his land so that they're actually respecting his identity.

The contrast between this and how government agencies have often operated is stark.

This crowd had been marshalled to come to Bourke and find out from the local community what they wanted in the way of alternative housing. So they found out … what the community had to say about the sorts of housing that would have been relevant to their needs as a community, and they went away and then a little while later they started building. They built these houses that were completely different to what the community had said that they wanted. And so they came back a little while later… to get some sort of an idea about further development of the housing projects that they might have been able to provide for the Bourke community. And the people were aghast and they said, "Well, why the hell should we tell you what we want when you've given us something which was completely different to what we last told you? We told you we wanted big houses with wide verandas to protect us from the sun and lots of big rooms in the house, even if there mightn't have been a whole lot of them, where you could have a lot of people in together because that's the way we are as a community. We want to be able to exist in the same room without all these little walls between us, and you've given us a house which is three by three."

Conclusion

John Gavaghan has maintained integrity and respect in the difficult and challenging areas related to child protection over a 40-year career in social work. He is driven by a commitment to diversity and respect and dignity for all people. He looks for ways that enhance human potential and for creative and innovative solutions to entrenched and intractable difficulties. He has had the benefit of a well-rounded education and has adopted a reflective approach to social work that has enabled him to continue to learn and develop while delivering services and programs in a collaborative and inclusive way. Well regarded by colleagues and people with whom he has worked, the summation of a group discussion of John Gavaghan was: "He is not cynical—he has worked with terrible painful humans who were doing terrible things to little children for 40 years and he is still committed, passionate, compassionate, interested, fascinated. He maintains a sense of humour and humility".

Chapter 6
What Can We Do to Make Changes?—Virginia (Ginni) Hall, AO

Emma Rush and A.W. (Bill) Anscombe

The faculty newsletter article written by proud colleague Paulene Curcuruto to celebrate Ginni's award of an Order of Australia Medal in 2014 describes Ginni as a "legend", but in conversation she is more likely to describe herself as a bit of a "ratbag". Her independence and dedicated engagement with issues that matter to her support both descriptions.

Born in Canberra in 1932, Ginni did not go to secondary school and initially trained as a nurse, specialising in obstetrics and infant welfare. She moved from nursing into social work through working with young people, first in the Girl Guides Association and then at McNally Training Centre, which was part of the juvenile justice system. She completed her Bachelor of Arts (Social Work) in Adelaide in her forties, and later completed both a postgraduate Diploma in Social Sciences and a Graduate Diploma of Education. For the last 25 years she has been associated with the School of Social Work and Community Welfare at James Cook University in Townsville, teaching and supervising fieldwork, but also undertaking important academic and professional leadership roles (including periods as both Head of Department and Associate Dean of the Faculty of Arts, Education and Social Sciences—and a period as the National President of the Australian Association of Social Work and Social Welfare Educators). She is now an adjunct staff member, but still supervises some student fieldwork.

Yet a great deal of Ginni's contribution has been through voluntary involvement with a range of community organisations. At the age of 82 she remains actively involved in eight different volunteer or community service groups (as she told the *Townsville Bulletin*, "It's just part of what I do"), and has recently been seen "flash mobbing" in shopping centres with a group she helped to found, Seniors Creating

E. Rush (✉) · A.W.(Bill) Anscombe
Charles Sturt University, Wagga Wagga, Australia
e-mail: erush@csu.edu.au

A.W.(Bill) Anscombe
e-mail: BAnscombe@csu.edu.au

M. Pawar et al. (eds.), *Empowering Social Workers*,
DOI 10.1007/978-981-10-3809-9_6

Change (see, for example, https://m.youtube.com/watch?v=U3feA7ILxjo). As the *Townsville Bulletin* article commemorating Ginni's receipt of her Order of Australia Medal put it, "retirement isn't on the horizon anytime soon" for Ginni. She is known for her independence and courage, her energy, dedication and resilience, and her resourcefulness, humanity and humility.

Biography

Early Life

Ginni was the only child of parents who both worked as public servants. Her parents' employment was particularly significant for Ginni in that it meant that her family moved from Canberra to Adelaide and then to Sydney, and finally to Brisbane, during her primary-school years. Over this period she attended *about six different schools*. The curriculum was different in each state, and as a result she was *put back* two years, finally finishing Grade 7 at boarding school, where she had been sent due to fears about the impact of the Second World War on Brisbane. By this time she was almost 14 and she decided to leave school. She followed in her mother's footsteps initially and *did shorthand and typing … and secretarial-type jobs*. She found that she didn't like this kind of work and when her parents, who *were having a lot of difficulties*, split up, she decided to follow her mother to Melbourne.

Nursing: "Really Loved … Working with People"

After they arrived in Melbourne, Ginni decided to train as a nurse, and this marked the beginning of the first, very significant, part of her working life. In due course it became evident that she *really loved* nursing, especially the *working with people* aspect, but she describes her immediate motivation as a very young woman as being much more pragmatic:

> I thought: Where's a job where I can get three meals a day, a roof over my head, and get some money, and do some work? … In those days [nurses] had to live in, you got fed, you got clothed, et cetera, and you got a pay packet of two pounds three and thruppence a fortnight.

Ginni proved to be very good at the medical as well as the "people" side of nursing, and won the surgical prize during her training at Prince Henry's Hospital in Melbourne. She went on to do her midwifery training at the Queen Victoria Hospital in Melbourne, and then her Certificate in Infant Welfare in Adelaide. She then took up a 12-month nursing position at Bordertown (in South Australia, but on the Victorian border) and while there made quite a remarkable decision.

> [O]ne of the women I was nursing with and myself, we said we need to do something different … what are we going to do with our lives? And so the pair of us applied for a job in Papua New Guinea. (Laughs) … And we both got a job up there. We both were sent to Port Moresby for three months, just to be … soaked up into the culture and educated, and all that sort of stuff. We worked in the Port Moresby Hospital. And [then] she got sent to one part of Papua New Guinea and I got sent to Madang, which was on the north coast of Papua New Guinea. And I was asked to set up a maternity ward, and a malnutrition babies' ward, and train women to become nurses. That was my job. (Laughs) … I loved my three years in Papua New Guinea, I really enjoyed it.

This impressive entry into the education of nurses—and Ginni's enthusiasm for teaching and her talent for it—meant that when she returned to South Australia in 1961 and applied for a position as the matron of Loxton Hospital. The selection committee there thought that Ginni *had a lot more skills and knowledge than I actually had!* But *it turned out really well.* She spent five years at Loxton, with continuing involvement in the training of nurses: *[W]e used to take training nurses for the first 12–18 months, and then transfer them to a hospital in Adelaide to finish their training so that they had that bigger experience, not just a country town.* Ginni also got involved in the community beyond the hospital while she was in Loxton—but not always in the way that the conservatism of the era appreciated!

> I played golf, and I played basketball, [which] was then known as men's basketball … But matrons of hospitals shouldn't be playing basketball. I was in trouble with the town because I was doing something that was rat baggy … [It was considered] totally inappropriate … As a matron … you know, you're supposed to set the role model … you're training those nurses too and you're just giving them a bad example … it was that period of time, mm … and it got even more reinforced because I broke my foot playing basketball and I was in a plaster cast for about five or six weeks. [They said] "See, told you so. [If you had] done as you [were] told … you wouldn't have that."

Youth Work: "If You Have the Right Sort of Relationship with Young People …"

Ginni became involved in youth work while in Loxton, particularly with the Girl Guides. When she decided to return to Adelaide she took up a 12-month "travelling trainer" position with the Girl Guides, which involved helping to develop their programs and setting up a Rangers unit for older girls. She enjoyed this work with young people and, although she continued to work in nursing for several more years (as deputy matron at Ashford Community Hospital, one of the then two private hospitals in Adelaide, from 1968 to 1970, and then on night shift while she completed a Certificate in Youth Work), this marked the beginning of a decisive shift in her career.

From 1971 until 1973 she held the position of matron/group worker at McNally Training Centre, which was part of the juvenile justice system, under the Department for Community Welfare. Although this was partly a nursing position,

Ginni also initiated the establishment of a community-based program for young offenders. She had become:

> very concerned about young people from rural areas at McNally, who every visiting day missed out on everything. Nothing happened [for them]. They were sitting around watching other people get visitors … So I got very political … I tried to negotiate with McNally Training Centre itself and couldn't get anywhere, so I went to the Minister. (Laughs). I didn't even know what I was doing in those days, I just did it. [I] said that I was concerned about young 14-, 15-year-old men, boys, being disadvantaged in terms of not having any access out in the community, and things like that. So he gave me permission each fortnight to take four boys out bushwalking, without a male staff member. (Laughs). Now these are young offenders by the way. And I used to take them down the kitchen, we'd cut lunch, then we'd go off bushwalking for a couple of hours in the Adelaide Hills and then come home again. Yeah. And that went on for two or three months. And then one day I think something happened, I can't remember, I got distracted or something like that, and when I went back looking for the boys they were missing. And I thought uh-oh, I've blown it. Anyway, the [bus] driver came to pick me up to take them back to McNally and you could see the big smirk on his face. (Laughs) You know exactly what I'm saying … And I thought oh well, I've blown it now, that it was worth trying but it didn't work. [But when I was dropped] back to McNally, [there were] the four boys standing at the front door of McNally knocking waiting to be let … asking to be let in. Because they had genuinely got lost, they'd got themselves a lift back to McNally, and one person you didn't abscond on was me … And so what I … gained out of that was you work well with people and give them some life opportunities and they will take notice of it and do something with it.

After Ginni left McNally, she worked at a youth project centre in Adelaide establishing a community-based program for young offenders. The program offered small group support, not counselling services, and it proved to be a very positive experience: *Some of those young offenders ended up being state footballers and all sorts of things*. This reinforced her experience at McNally that, when offered appropriate support, people can change their lives radically for the better.

> It's something I lived with for many years thinking, "You can do it, you can do it." … [I]f you have the right sort of relationship with young people you can get them to that." Students often say to me, "What's the difference between social work and psychology?" And I say, "Psychologists see the problem in the person; social workers see a problem in the environment in which the person has to manage their life."

Social Work and Social-Work Education: "Interacting with Students"

While Ginni was completing her Certificate in Youth Work, the teaching staff had repeatedly said to her, *Why don't you do social work? (Laughs). Why don't you do social work?* She commenced studying part time for her social work degree at the South Australian Institute of Technology. While studying, she held the position of Director of Consultation and Training at the Services to Youth Council in Adelaide, and then in the middle years of her degree she moved to the University of Adelaide as a student counsellor. In the final years of her degree she obtained a position as a lecturer in social work at the South Australian Institute of Technology. When she had completed her degree, an opportunity came up to go and work in Indonesia for a year, under the auspices of the Hawthorn Institute of Education in Melbourne (later absorbed into the University of Melbourne).

> So I thought why not. I've worked in Papua New Guinea, I could work in Indonesia, [I] can't speak the language but it doesn't matter. [The position] was to work with the Schools of Social Work in Indonesia to help them upgrade their curriculum, make it more relevant for their community and their structure, and their society. And so I spent a year … living in Jakarta, just travelling around Indonesia visiting Schools of Social Work in Indonesia, helping them restructure and rewrite their curriculum. I mean it wasn't quite the same as [social work] down here [in Australia], but it was [similar enough] … so yeah, that was an exciting year as you can well imagine.

When she returned to Australia she continued to work with the Hawthorn Institute of Education, as the Coordinator of Fellowship and Welfare Services. This position involved:

> working with students from overseas, encouraging and supporting them and developing their skills … During that period also they sent me to Fiji for three months to develop youth work programs for Fiji. So I'm getting a lot of introduction to … different cultural backgrounds and things like that, even if I didn't speak the language. (Laughs).

Then a position came up at James Cook University in Townsville. Ginni made a *very deliberate* decision to apply: *I want(ed) to go and live in a smaller community where I could have more contact with people and … be involved in things happening in the community.* Ginni was appointed as a lecturer and commenced in 1988. She progressed to senior lecturer, and held various leadership positions: Head of Department of Social Work and Community Welfare (1994–1996); Director of Centre for Women's Studies (1996–1999) and Associate Dean of the Faculty of Arts, Education and Social Sciences (1998–1999). She remains an adjunct senior lecturer, supervising student fieldwork, which she loves. Ginni chose not to pursue a research path, and her academic career has been strongly practice and education based:

> It just didn't mean a lot to me to sit down and spend months writing on a piece of paper. For me personally, I was much more, and still am, much more interested in interacting with students, talking with them: what are you doing and what are you learning, how are you making sense of that for yourself, how are you making sense of that for your client, what would … if you saw that client again in that situation would you do the same thing, or would you do it differently? If so, why? So … that's my framework.

Volunteering: "It Gives My Head a Wider Picture of the Community"

In over 25 years since she went to live in Townsville, Ginni's initial desire *to be involved in things happening in the community* has been fulfilled to such an extent that when her colleagues in the voluntary sector nominated her for an Order of

Australia Medal they commenced the nomination with: "[S]he has become an icon within the Townsville Welfare sector". The nomination form records Ginni's "cheerfulness and willingness to contribute to her community", and notes that "due to her depth of knowledge and experience, Governments seek Ginni out to undertake a range of roles that supports the most disadvantaged within our community".

Extraordinary as it may sound, since she has been in Townsville Ginni has been involved, and in many cases very substantially involved, in *eighteen* different community initiatives in Townsville and North Queensland. These range from representing her community on government commissions, tribunals and community forums, to volunteering at Reef HQ aquarium, where she still *talk[s] to the fish* every Monday morning, and encourages *people visiting Townsville … to think about the reef, to think about conservation, to think about the damage that can be done or has been done to the reef, to think about climate change*. Her current (2014) commitments also include one day a week volunteering with the Townsville Community Information Centre, half a day a week volunteering at the World Vision shop, regular letter writing and sit-ins with Amnesty International, and participation on a range of committees: Everglow (previously Ethnic) Community Care Links (of which she is currently the president); Althea Projects (previously Wee Care Family); Queensland Youth Services; Townsville Legal Service Elder Abuse Committee; Domestic Violence Resource Service and the Feminist Collective.

More broadly, while in Townsville, the areas Ginni has been involved in (including those she remains in) in a voluntary/community service capacity include: community health, legal aid, women's services, family and children's services, youth services, aged care, electoral reform, community housing, Indigenous issues, international development and justice, and environmental initiatives. It is hardly surprising that the nomination for Ginni's Order of Australia Medal states emphatically: "Ginni goes wherever she is needed! Her time, skills and commitment have, over many years, had an enormous benefit to all the worthy causes she is involved in".

Ginni herself notes:

> [W]hen I was younger I never thought I would be doing [volunteering], I mean that just didn't even enter my perspective … [but] volunteering has become a really important part of my life [and because] it's not all the same sort of organisation or same place … it gives my head a wider picture of the community.

It seems fitting to close Ginni's biography to this point with an insight into one of the causes she is currently involved in and *very passionate about*. It is also particularly topical, given the demographic changes confronting Australia.

> It's a group of seniors [people over the age of 50 years, from diverse religious and ethnic backgrounds, including myself] that got together about three years ago saying: 'We're not happy with a lot of the things that are happening with the seniors in this community, what can we do to make changes?'

With the support of the Townsville Community Legal Service, *we put together this choir, [called] Seniors Creating Change*.

> [W]e go all over the place entertaining elders, singing songs. A lot of our songs are human rights or social justice type songs, and quite a few of the members are social workers … it's one of my passions, every Saturday morning is choir … It's not even so much the singing, it's the choir … [W]e started off with about 15 people, the choir now has about 60 in it, and on any Saturday morning, normally at least about 40 turn up. And that means that a whole lot of seniors who are isolated or lonely come … and reach out. I pick up two and bring them to the choir' cause they don't get out of the house other than this trip on Saturday mornings. So that's… it's a social event for them as well as we get out there and thump the table… it definitely has a political bias to it … "If I Had a Hammer" is one of our very popular ones. We do that as a flash mob. Now seniors aren't flash mobbing, they don't flash mob. It's teenagers who flash mob. So we go to Woolworths here in town and sit around in the café and somebody stands up and says, "If I had a hammer," and somebody else responds to that, and then we all stand up and take our [over]shirts off [to show our Seniors Creating Change tee-shirts underneath] and start singing. And … Woolworths love it.

> [O]n Elder Abuse Day each year we now take to the streets and march … what we're doing with this is acknowledging elder abuse and getting people to think about it and question it and stuff like that … the Townsville Community Legal Service sees at least 40 cases [of elder abuse, predominantly financial abuse] a month.

The World Health Organization describes elder abuse as follows: "Elder abuse is a violation of human rights and a significant cause of injury, illness, lost productivity, isolation and despair" (WHO 2002, *Active Ageing, A Policy Framework*, p. 29).

In 2013, with the support of the Townsville Community Legal Service, a small booklet describing the work of Seniors Creating Change was produced. It emphasised that "ageism is at the heart of many seniors' issues" and highlighted the importance of "positive ageing", noting that the group's "work as positive role models can only become more important as time goes by" (Mitchell 2013, p. 15; p. 14). It highlighted the various aims of the group, including to empower the seniors involved to "raise awareness of issues affecting seniors" and to "sing for justice, freedom, respect and dignity" (Mitchell 2013, p. 7).

Theme song: When the Seniors Create Change (Tune: When the Saints Come Marching In)

Individual voices:
We are travelling in the footsteps

of those who've gone before
and we will stand united
until a new world is in store
some people say this ageist world
is the only one we need
but we're waiting for that morning

ALL: When a new world is revealed.
ALL:
We are the seniors creating change, we are the seniors creating change
Oh how I want to be in that number, when the seniors create change.
[And so on, until the final stanza as follows]
We are the seniors creating change, we are the seniors creating change
We want YOU to be in that number, and we ALL can create change.

To see a full performance, visit: https://www.youtube.com/watch?v=-es1aLGdu9Y

Analysis of Qualities/Character

It is evident for many people that their positive character traits or virtues originated in early direct influences from their family, schooling or religion, but Ginni did not identify these as significant influences for her. Rather, she comments that some of her values, such as a commitment to international justice, *over time I've developed myself.* Moreover, she notes that some of her commitments have become more explicit and refined over time. For example, when she worked in Papua New Guinea (1959–1961, before the successes of civil rights movements in the 1960s), the hospitals were segregated by race. Ginni was the only fully trained nurse in the "black hospital" and she was confined to the maternity and malnutrition babies ward, although there were also local women assisting in the hospital who had had some nursing training. In contrast, there were five trained nurses in the "white hospital", which was much smaller. Ginni recalls that at the time she did not really think in terms of racism or equality. *I just thought: well this is what's happening, what do we do about it?... [T]he racism issue I probably didn't think of or even understand all that well at that stage. But as I grew up I did.* She concludes that both circumstances and reflective practice have probably influenced the development of her character over time.

Independence and Courage

One of the virtues that stands out most strongly in the story of Ginni's life is independence. Ginni herself reflects that this may have partly been developed as a result of her particular childhood: an only child, *so from that perspective I was probably a little bit independent doing things for myself*, and one who *moved on all the time* due to parental work commitments, meaning *I didn't make any long-term friends.* It is hardly surprising that she mentions that in her final years of school (late childhood to early adolescence) she enjoyed the experience of boarding school, and also notes enjoying her later experience of living in the nurses' home while she did her nursing training.

However, even if developed under somewhat adverse conditions, this independence stood her in extremely good stead when she developed her career. She comments *when [an] opportunity comes up I go with it.* This was illustrated perhaps most clearly in her decision to apply for the position in Papua New Guinea while still very early in her career, but it reappears time and time again in her long and varied working life, including in her voluntary and community service commitments. In a number of examples from Ginni's life story, her independence is accompanied by courage, which manifests most clearly when it involves challenging powerful structures that prevent properly respecting and caring for people.

Both independence and courage are highlighted in a story of principled resistance against corporate power from her time in Papua New Guinea (1959–1961).

> Nestlé sent me a cargo ship, one of those huge big things, of powdered milk. I went how good is that, we received all this powdered milk to come to mothers who have no sense of hygiene, no sense of washing, no sense of boiling water, no sense of even measuring things etc. … And so I had to go through a whole political thing of putting that cargo back and sending it back to Brisbane. (laughs) So I did get politically involved in doing things even then even though I didn't really understand that's what I was doing. Yeah [there] was just no way this milk is going to stay in this town under any circumstances … Put it back on the ship and send it back, yep (laugh). So there is a slightly proactive sort of (laugh)… You know break the rules when you can.

Ginni's efforts to take the young offenders from McNally bushwalking is a similar example of principled challenging of the system. She has never broken rules for no reason, but she is not inclined to accept established boundaries for which there are no good reasons (her playing of what was then called "men's basketball" in Loxton is one example of this), and she recognises that there are times when a little bit of the "ratbag" is needed to achieve important social goals. It is also important to remember that balancing Ginni's independence is a very strong capacity to work with others, as is amply demonstrated by her life's work.

Ginni notes that freedom from family responsibilities meant that unlike many women, she was able to retain her independence throughout her working life. She did not marry ["I was engaged twice, but one went and got himself killed in an aeroplane and the other one turned gay (laughs)"] nor have children, and both her parents died in their early 60s, *when I was only in the early part of my career … So I mean I have really lived my life with me being in control of it … I've been able to make my own choices and own decisions.*

Energy, Dedication and Resilience

Even in her retirement, Ginni's life is very visibly one of energy and engagement. She is a *doer*: someone who *does* things (rather than simply thinking or talking about them)—and she doesn't stop until she finishes the thing she has set out to do. Much social work training now focuses on reflective practice and articulating conflicts, but Ginni's own training in nursing, youth work and social work would have been very practically focused. The sheer number and range of Ginni's achievements in her working life (both in a paid and a voluntary capacity) testify that she has an inspirational capacity to stick at work she considers important. Getting the unwanted powdered milk back onto the ship and bound for Brisbane is just one example from her early career in Papua New Guinea; starting a bush-walking program for the young inhabitants of the McNally Training Centre in South Australia is another. A number of Ginni's colleagues recognised her dedication in their letters of support for her Order of Australia Medal, with Marsha Davies (CEO, Coast to Country Housing) highlighting Ginni's "dedication" and "diligence" (Curcuruto 2014).

Ginni herself notes of her nursing training: *It was very, very disciplined in those days. And at one level I think it was probably good for me. (laughs) I mean I probably didn't see it as that [at the time], but [it was] very disciplined.* She agrees that discipline can achieve things that wouldn't have been achieved otherwise.

The longevity of Ginni's commitment to working for a better world speaks also to her resilience: her capacity to sustain dedication under adverse conditions. When queried about how she continues her work in difficult times—a regular challenge for social workers—Ginni commented as follows:

> One of the tough things that I have had happen is I have had breast cancer and had to deal with that and I had to go through all the dramas of chemotherapy and radiotherapy and all that sort of stuff, but I kept coming to work and I kept being focused on getting on with life and doing things, not letting it take over my life. So I think it's that sort of thing and … yeah … maybe that's because I think I have something to contribute (chuckle). I mean that sounds a bit… have you got something to contribute have you? Aren't you lucky? But I mean I think the background I've had, the sort of life I've had, I do have some things to contribute to the community and I have a right and a responsibility to see that I share those with the community.

Along with a firm grip on the bigger picture and a sense of the importance of giving back as just described, Ginni also says that *put[ting] behind you what you've been doing during the day* in order to avoid the occupational hazards of stress and burn-out is *really, really important but not easy*. Different things work for different people.

> I've got good next door neighbours and most afternoons when I go home I go next door and have a beer with them or a glass of wine and chat for half an hour but nothing to do with work and by the time I go back inside work's gone and I'm watching telly and doing other things (laughs) … that's how I do it for me.

Finally, she describes herself as *an optimist rather than a pessimist*. This may be another of the keys to sustaining dedication—optimism within the bounds of what is realistically likely to be possible in the short to medium term:

> I would probably say I can't fix the world but there are things that I can do on a day-to-day basis or on a weekly basis or in sitting down with students and working with them that can change a small part in somebody's life that they choose to have changed that makes it better for them.

Her letter writing for Amnesty International provides a good example of this optimism (and also shows her challenging powerful structures):

> [W]e have what we call letter writing night once a month where [we have several reports of] things that have been happening, not just in Australia but around the world, and we sit down as a group and write letters to the Prime Ministers or the Presidents or whoever of those countries and challenge them about how a particular situation is being handled and ask them to consider doing it differently and make some suggestions of how that could happen. And we do that the first Wednesday of every month, we sit down and do letter writing, yeah. And I probably get three, four, sometime five letters a year back. Not that many but at least you get some response. And others get response back occasionally too. So we're making… at least people stop and think. We're not saying they're changing their behaviour or anything like that but at least if we get them to stop and think, maybe over

time they might sort of say maybe we can do this differently … And I mean I know that there are times where nothing will change, I mean I accept that, it's the reality of life but if you don't do something then nobody even gets questioned or challenged.

Resourcefulness

Resourcefulness is the capacity for creativity with scarce resources. It is a perennially useful quality for social workers, who frequently face constrained resources for the task at hand, and it has enabled Ginni's independence and dedication to be fully effective in achieving what she set out to do throughout her long career. It is also a quality that would have been regularly practised during Ginni's early childhood in the Depression years: "gumption" (shrewd or spirited initiative and resourcefulness) was a quality highly prized in that era.

A story from her early nursing work in Papua New Guinea illustrates Ginni's resourcefulness beautifully.

[W]e didn't have a [regular] doctor [in the "black hospital"] so I was it. So a mother had her baby and the baby lived or died on the basis of my knowledge and what I did, and I used to have real—this was a fun thing—rules for the mothers. What I was about was them not going home until their breast milk was well established so I had to work out a way of doing that. And I thought how do I do that because they won't understand what I'm talking about with their breast milk coming [Ginni could not speak the local language to that level of complexity] but the cord on the baby's tummy I used to strap it on and say you can't go home until "The rope belong piccaninny go finish" … In other words until the baby's cord has dropped off you can't go home. And we used to stick it on the extra two or three days and it meant two or three more days of establishing mum's milk and getting her organised so that by the time she went home… (laughs) there was a very good chance of that baby surviving because there was sufficient breast milk.

Humanity/Compassion

Concern for humanity, the importance for all people of *[j]ust being treated as a person, just being treated as an individual who has an opportunity to do something*, shines strongly in not only what Ginni has chosen to do in her life, but in the way that she has done it. In her letter of support for Ginni's Order of Australia Medal nomination, Anita Berry (Manager of Volunteering North Queensland) describes her as a "humanitarian in the true spirit of the word" (Curcuruto 2014). Queried over where she might have developed this virtue, Ginni reflects: *[A]t one level I probably thought I was a bit less fortunate than other people, I suspect, you know, the fact that I'd spent a bit of time … in different places myself … that might have been it.* She didn't have a strong religious background, and although she had a Catholic education for some parts of her schooling, she does not credit it with a strong influence in this way: *[R]eligion and church itself has not ever been a priority in my life, but some of the concepts that they talk about in terms of caring for people … that certainly does [count as a priority in my life], yeah.*

One example from Ginni's current community service activity with Amnesty International underlines her sense of this humanity/compassion in terms it is difficult to ignore.

> The first Friday every month at 8am we [Amnesty International members] stand outside Ewen Jones', who is our Federal Member's, office for half an hour and challenge him about the way the Government is treating refugees. They're not being respected, they're not being treated appropriately, they're being sent back to where they came from and I've done quite a lot of research and reading about refugees and one of my heartfelt concerns is the kids. What kids are seeing happening to their families and to themselves, what kids are being taught to do. I talked to a mother here five or six years ago now and I said to her: Why did you have to leave your home town? She said: Because my son was being taught how to use a gun and I had to leave, I could not have my seven-year-old boy being shown how to use a rifle or a gun and to use it on somebody else. He wasn't just being shown how to use a gun but it was to [be] used on somebody else. You know that sort of stuff. I guess that pushes buttons inside me and I say … you know, that's not what this world should be about.

It is not *what this world should be about*, and that Ginni still engages in such civil action in her eighties also shows that her challenging of powerful structures that prevent properly respecting and caring for people is still going strong. She notes that when humanity/compassion is linked to social work's understanding of structural problems, it can make a real difference in helping to empower people to make positive changes in their own lives:

> [A social work client] may have to do some sorting out of themselves, but a lot of it is due to the pressures that the external environment is putting on them that means that they have difficulties in that area. And you know, students' eyes light up when I say that. "Oh, yeah." It's sort of, mm, they can see the point of [seeing the person within the structures, rather than seeing the person as the problem].

Humility

Ginni's first reaction to the news of her nomination for an Order of Australia was reportedly "surprise and amazement"; "She could not understand why she was nominated" (Curcuruto 2014). Humility tends to be illustrated most strongly by what a person doesn't say—as well as how they say what they do say. Ginni brushes off the description of her as a "legend", which opened this chapter, with the claim that the colleague who wrote that description was just *being nice*. But her colleagues across the board would clearly differ from her on this. In their submissions in support of her award of an Order of Australia Medal, "humility" is explicitly identified as one of Ginni's valued qualities (Marsha Davies, CEO, Coast to Country Housing) and she is described as "self-effacing" and a "quiet achiever" (Anita Berry, Manager of Volunteering North Queensland). But her colleagues are very clear that she is a "much loved person and very well respected amongst her peers" (Deanne Bell, retired City Councillor, Townsville).

Humility seems an underrated virtue in the current era, when social expectations—and especially social media—encourage making much of oneself, no matter how insignificant the details of one's life are. Humility leads away from this encouragement of putting the self at the centre of the picture, and Ginni is very clear about its importance at the core of social work.

> Occasionally with some students I may even ask them: why did you decide to do social work? … I mean there are some students that I've actually encouraged to… [g]o in another direction … they're not going to be all that good to work with clients anyway … They don't listen to people, they don't pay attention, their priorities are first, it's about me not you… Me, me, me, me …

Conclusion

Of her long career and involvement in community service activities, Ginni says:

> If I had a choice to do it again, yes I would because I think that if I have some understanding and some knowledge of the world and the environment and the dynamics of what's happening, including the political agenda, which is going on the whole time and the impact that that has on agencies, communities and individuals, if I can make a small change to help one person negotiate that drama, great.

Ginni embodies core qualities of the social work profession: independence and courage, compassion and humanity, energy, dedication and resilience. Some of Ginni's other character traits, developed during a very different era from the present one, are qualities that are now perhaps seen less in social work, but from which we might draw inspiration and seek to develop more in the profession: resourcefulness and humility.

In any life, but particularly a life as full of engagement as Ginni's, it is inevitable that a very great deal will be left out in the attempt to capture a chapter-length sketch of it. Those who nominated Ginni for the Order of Australia noted in the nomination that they were aware that "we may not know the full extent of the many layers of community interests that Ginni becomes involved in, and the full extent of the impact of her work". We can only hope to have captured some of the essentials here, and we acknowledge that much has necessarily been left out.

References

Curcuruto, P. (2014, 30 January). OAM anyone? *SASS News*, School of Arts and Social Sciences, James Cook University, Townsville, p. 2.

Mitchell, B. (2013). *Seniors creating change: From idea to intervention*. Townsville Community Legal Service Inc.

Chapter 7
A People World, Rather Than a Paper World—Bronwyn Hyde

Manohar Pawar and Wendy Bowles

At the time of interview, Bronwyn Hyde was the Senior Social Worker, Mental Health, at Orange Health Service in rural New South Wales. She graduated in social work in 1976 from the University of Sydney and commenced work in rural NSW with the fledgling Community Health Services, as one of two social workers within a multidisciplinary team. After gaining a diploma in education, Bronwyn was employed in the TAFE system for some years within the child studies and community services sectors, firstly as a part-time teacher and then as a full-time teacher and acting head teacher. She then returned to social work in 2001, securing a position with a child and adolescent mental health team working across both hospital and community settings in Orange. During this time she attained a Graduate Diploma in Mental Health (Child and Adolescent) from the Institute of Psychiatry, before completing her Master of Social Work (Advanced Practice) at Charles Sturt University in 2009.

Prior to her return to social work in Australia Bronwyn worked as a social worker in a culturally diverse area of East London, for Newham Social Services, in the field of child protection. She is currently enrolled in the Doctor of Social Work course through Charles Sturt University and is completing her research on recovery-oriented practice within a rural mental health inpatient facility. Her thesis is entitled "The lived experience of an admission to a mental health inpatient unit—what's recovery got to do with it?" Bronwyn's life and practice suggests to emphatically refocus on basics: deep listening, relationship building, locating in the people world and questioning the "taken for granted" assumptions.

M. Pawar (✉) · W. Bowles
School of Humanities and Social Sciences, Charles Sturt University,
Wagga Wagga, Australia
e-mail: mpawar@csu.edu.au

W. Bowles
e-mail: wbowles@csu.edu.au

M. Pawar et al. (eds.), *Empowering Social Workers*,
DOI 10.1007/978-981-10-3809-9_7

Birth and Early Parental and Family Influences

Bronwyn Hyde was born in 1953, the youngest of three children, with an older sister and brother. Her father and uncle were school teachers, her mother had been a midwife and nurse before she got married and started the family. In those days women had no choice about combining career and raising a family—if they wanted to marry and have children they had to give up their jobs and become stay-at-home mothers. Bronwyn grew up in Bexley North, looking over the Bardwell Valley towards the city, in what is now known as the inner south-western suburbs of Sydney.

The first thing that comes to Bronwyn's mind about her early life is her family's strong emphasis on academic achievement:

> Not that it was overt I suppose … it was just something that you picked up … and our achievements at school were greatly celebrated and encouraged … we probably got most of our encouragement from Mum.

Bronwyn's mother had a strong love of learning that persists into later life (she was still learning French in her middle nineties). Bronwyn recalls getting teased about the lengths her mother would go to in getting background research to help with primary school projects. Both Bronwyn and her sister wanted to do well for their parents and to gain their approval—the excitement of celebrating his children's achievements is one of the few times that Bronwyn remembers her usually reserved father being demonstrative. For Bronwyn, being the youngest in the family meant being the observer: *I just sat back ... and watched the family unfold before me, and learnt from it*. Instead of openly rebelling against her parents and their values, as her brother and sister had done, Bronwyn chose a different strategy:

> So I kept out of it, kept things to myself and it probably worked for mum and dad too that … they didn't have to deal with it all the time. … I didn't want to hurt them and I didn't want to have to be confronted with all that difference either so I just left home quietly and [laughing] got on with things that I knew they wouldn't want me to be doing.

Schooling and Further Education—Choice of Social Work

Primary school was a wonderful time in Bronwyn's life—she made lifelong friends and is still in touch with people from primary-school days, despite the group scattering to different high schools for their secondary schooling. Having her uncle, with whom she was very close, as her sixth-grade teacher and deputy principal of the primary school *cements me to that experience I suppose*.

Primary school was the first time that Bronwyn became aware that not everyone had the same advantages of growing up in a stable, happy home with two *parents that loved me*. Boys from the Salvation Army Boys' Home also attended the school and Bronwyn was acutely aware of their difference from the other children—from the smell of their Brylcreemed hair to noticing *a roughness and sadness* about their situation. Bronwyn remembers inviting two of them to her birthday party as *that kind of need to include them in something that was normal and warm and friendly and yeah, family oriented ... Maybe that's where it all came from.*

Looking back, Bronwyn thinks that her focus on relationships is the thing that really influenced her decision to go into social work *and probably sustained me there.* Explaining this emphasis on relationships Bronwyn comments: *I don't have what I would call a huge social network but I've got intense special friends that have been with me for a long time and I think that's how I like to be. I have those very close friendships.*

Another strong influence in Bronwyn's choice of social work was the social upheaval going on at the time, *a strong influence of feminism, you could feel that coming through* … and *questioning things that our parents just took for granted.* She said:

> the 60s and the moratorium of Vietnam and the flower power and all those traditional values that we'd been raised on in the 50s and 60s absolutely being shattered. And I often think how challenging it must have been for our parents who grew up in a very different mindset—having children now grow up in this society and world that was just so far removed from all the values that they had been raised with and that they had thought they had imbued us with as well.

While Bronwyn's elder sister went into medicine, psychiatry and later became a professor of medicine, her brother took the opposite path of *drugs, sex and rock and roll.* This meant, in Bronwyn's eyes, that there was no option left for her, or rather only the choice of what to study at university:

> And I really don't know how social work came on the agenda. I can't remember why necessarily I went down that path, except for one thing that I remember thinking: I've had such a fortunate life I would like to be able to help others who haven't had such a fortunate life. So that was I think, probably the only rationale that I remember making in that decision to pursue social work.

Although her first two university years were lonely, Bronwyn appreciated the *wide view* afforded by introductory subjects (anthropology, psychology and education) and *the opportunity to play around them.* Third year was the beginning of social work itself, a significant change in focus, which meant that many people dropped out. Bronwyn attributes this self-selection partly to the confronting nature of *the very strong focus on your own self-learning, self-development.* She herself found the last two years at university, the Whitlam years, to be *a very inspiring time to be in social work.*

Two things stand out for Bronwyn from these two years—feminism and learning the art of listening. A fellow student inspired her to learn and read about feminism—it is to his influence that Bronwyn attributes her shift away from her parents' traditional values, and her desire to not be a married, stay-at-home mother. The other big step at this time was learning how difficult the art of listening is—*discovering the difference between wanting to fix and allowing a solution to emerge … It was one of those light bulb "ah ha" moments where I realised there was so much power in doing what felt like a whole lot less but in fact was really difficult and crucial to your empowering kind of relationship with somebody.*

Bronwyn learnt her feminism and the art of listening at a personal as well as a political level; this experiential learning *was a real eye opener for me as a person as well ... I don't think any other course I did at uni would have resulted in those two kinds of changes, shifts in being, in a sense of self, like they did.*

Trained in community development and group work and completing two placements in local councils in communities awash with money from the Australian Assistance Plan, Bronwyn graduated with the understanding that her purpose was *to change the world.* However, at the same time she wondered if she *had the conviction to do that.* She puts this lack of conviction down to two issues: first, a lack of confidence to be a political activist leader and second, the ability to see several sides of an issue. She comments:

> I think this comes from being able to see too many points of view and finding it hard to settle on one absolutely that would then become my "mission". I also always doubt that I know enough about a particular issue or fear that I'm being one-sided to the exclusion of other viewpoints. The postmodern dilemma!

Social Work Practice Career

On graduation and following her childhood dream to live in the country, Bronwyn moved to Bathurst in regional New South Wales and visited the new community health centre, or polyclinic as it was called, to ask about work: *I remember walking in asking ... about what work was available and within a couple of weeks I had a letter saying congratulations you start on such and such a day. I didn't go in for an interview—I went into just enquire.*

These were the first heady days of community health, with a strong emphasis on community development and prevention. There were plenty of resources for staff, who were all trying to create new community-based roles outside of hospital—whether they were experienced nurses or newly graduated social workers or psychologists. It is important to Bronwyn that her early days in social work were imbued with a positive health focus rather than ill health: *our mission was to prevent ill health, not just to work with those who were already feeling poorly emotionally or physically.*

However, Bronwyn also remembers the clear status divisions between *professionals* and nurses at the polyclinic: professionals got a big car, a Falcon, and nurses got a little car, an Escort. However, by choice Bronwyn opted for a nice little Escort and still remembered its number: *HSW 160 ... I used to think it stood for Hotshot Social Worker.*

Bronwyn remembers the developing team, united by their mission to pioneer community health, forging relationships in other departments and services; how team members became firm friends, socialising outside work hours as well as being colleagues at work. There was a sense of experimentation; running an evening group on head lice and how to prevent it with the community nurse wasn't something that was taught at university. Working with clergy and local government departments, Bronwyn and her colleagues established a 24-h Lifeline counselling service in Bathurst and Orange, training the volunteers and getting the service going. This was a happy time, with young, single team members and more *motherly*, older nurses—*they were a nice balance to us young ones.*

The interprofessional focus of her work is one of the advantages of rural and regional life, according to Bronwyn. In contrast to her city-based colleagues, she and other health workers joined forces with GPs, child protection welfare officers and social security staff through interagency and other groups right from the beginning: *we had this wonderful working mindset... around we're all in it together, we're all going to help*. She was surprised during a meeting in Sydney to discover that city-based health social work was much more siloed in comparison, and only just beginning to think about working with other services and departments.

Within the first 12 months Bronwyn was appointed team leader, a job she took on with enthusiasm, even though *looking back I think oh how could I have had the skills, the experience to really take that on?* From 1976 to 1979, when she left work to have her first baby, Bronwyn remained team leader. This meant she co-ordinated and managed community health staff, as well as developing and presenting health education programs and providing casework to individuals and families.

She attributes her early leadership appointment partly to the privileging of professionals over nurses noted above, as well as the Director *seeing something in me*. One of the things she feels she has missed in her career is the benefit of mentors and experienced social workers as models for practice. Instead, in her first year out of university she was the role model: *became the senior social worker way before my time I think.* In testament to the professionalism of her team, Bronwyn comments that it was not till years later that she learnt that some of the older, more experienced nurses resented this young professional being appointed as team leader. One nurse was even inspired to enrol in a Masters degree in order to become a manager, having seen Bronwyn's early promotion.

A strong memory is the way *the whole place fell apart* when the administrative staff refused to make tea and the ritual of gathering for shared morning tea stopped —how important this was for team dynamics. *We all realised the importance when it was no longer happening*. Despite these ups and downs and various professional disciplines asserting themselves in different ways, the team spirit persisted, with five- and ten-year reunions attended by not only team members, but the Director and Deputy Director of Health, right up until their deaths in recent years. Even in their 80s and 90s these directors would attend the reunions: *That's how close not just our little team in the polyclinic was but the whole concept of community health they felt responsible for as well.*

The Department of Health provided two senior social workers, who were responsible for social work services across New South Wales: Lindsey Napier and Pam Burridge. They flew out from Sydney every few months to provide group supervision for all the social workers in the Bathurst-Orange area, including the social worker at the Department of Social Security. Bronwyn deeply appreciated how they connected to and supported social workers.

Negotiating Work and Family

While she was working at Bathurst Bronwyn married her husband, a nurse, who had two daughters from a previous marriage. Much to her own mother's surprise, within the first 12 months Bronwyn was pregnant and had three daughters in quick succession during the next three and a half years. The two daughters from her husband's first marriage lived with their mother during school term and with their father and Bronwyn for school holidays: *all five girls see themselves as sisters—no "half" about it. I think I have been very blessed to have this extended family.*

Bronwyn and her husband moved to Orange, another regional town only 50 kilometres from Bathurst, where housing was cheaper and he was already working. An equivalent position in Orange community health soon became available for Bronwyn. Like Bathurst, the team at community health in Orange was young and predominantly women.

Despite the story in Bathurst and Orange that regional towns are conservative and difficult to break into, Bronwyn didn't find it difficult at all. In fact: *We had a lovely time, now as a married couple. And then having babies.* Her personal relationships continued to develop from her work relationships, *and I think that's still the case.*

While the close and co-operative working environment and community were some of the advantages of being in a regional community, Bronwyn also recognises the disadvantages, although these haven't been too much of a problem for her. Things like choosing not to enrol in a Tai Chi class because she knew a client would be there, or deciding not to help in the new family business—a newsagency—in order to protect both herself and her clients. After working behind the counter for a couple of years, she decided to stop that when she returned to social work, putting herself into her clients' shoes and imagining what it would be like if someone she was seeing professionally walked into the newsagency:

> if I had just exposed myself with a revelation of, for example sexual assault as a child and it was the first time I'd ever revealed that and we were working on that together. And then I'd walk into the local newsagency and find that same person selling me a lottery ticket. I think I'd be devastated.

Bronwyn was determined not to be a stay-at-home mother. During the period when her three daughters were little she worked in various short-term, part-time and casual capacities, running parent groups or other educational groups in Health, and taking part-time teaching roles at TAFE. Another advantage of living in a rural community, Bronwyn feels, is your profile: *You don't get forgotten so easily so*

I would be often called on ... asked if I wanted to do this part-time work or casual work.

During this time Bronwyn began to realise how transferrable her social work skills are, in preventative and educative roles where a community development focus and group work skills are useful. TAFE started to offer her more work in the faculty of child studies, teaching communication and interpersonal skills subjects.

> I love that sharing of knowledge ... experiential learning... providing opportunities for people to experience things... seeing people change and become aware of certain aspects around themselves and the way that they related to others. I really enjoyed that so I thought no, maybe teaching is something I'd really like to do.

In 1986 a short stint at the Department of Social Security convinced Bronwyn that she didn't want to work there long term, although she did learn a great deal. She was impressed by the power to help or hinder that social workers wielded, and shocked at the differences in organisational culture between Health and Social Security—the way one worker was allowed to insult another during meetings with no rebuke from managers present: *I'm sure it does happen in other settings ... but ... it was a shock that people didn't have a basic understanding of boundaries and appropriateness.*

Return to Study and TAFE Teaching, 1987–1993

When the girls were around three, five and six years old, and with the support *of a wonderful husband who looked after those little ones all the time I was doing that,* Bronwyn decided to pursue the educational side of her interests. In 1987 she enrolled in a Graduate Diploma in Education in infants primary teaching (known as a Dip. Ed.) by distance education through Armidale College of Advanced Education. She *absolutely loved the study*. Every aspect of this course was a pleasure: the residential schools held two or three times a year, meeting fellow students and the two stints of prac teaching. Bronwyn was delighted to find that studying child development when her own children were little meant the content of her studies *was happening right in front of me*. She even enjoyed what would be a gruelling study regime to other people, fitting in study with part-time teaching at TAFE and raising three small children:

> We'd get dinner on the table, kids bathed, into bed, I would get all my books out, and then I would fall asleep in front of the telly with the books all around me. I'd have an hour or so sleep in front of the telly and then around 11 o'clock I'd wake up, and I'd study until about two o'clock in the morning. House was quiet. It was wonderful. So I'd have the peace and quiet to study and then go to bed about two o'clock, and have four hours, five hours sleep and then get up ... And then I got into that routine of sleeping between about 10 and 12 or 9 and 11 or something like that and then studying into the early hours of the morning.

Bronwyn finished her two-year diploma in 1988. She smiles at her response to her success:

> I won the College Medal and I didn't know that I had won the College Medal and it was at graduation and my name was … I was wondering why I was at the front of the queue because I'm H and I should have been back, and they announced my name and said I'd won the College Medal.

Although she enjoyed her studies and prac teaching, Bronwyn never worked as a school teacher. Instead she applied her learning from both her social work and Dip. Ed. to teaching adults in the Diploma of Community Services (Child Studies) in child development and social science subjects. She remained in part-time teaching positions at the Orange TAFE campus till 1993. Bronwyn notes that her group work and her listening skills are especially important in her teaching:

> I still think they're [skills] just as important in an educational sense as they are in the social work sense … the being able to know where somebody is at, to really be listening and be able to listen on a group level and to get people discussing with each other rather than have me as the focal point and all those kinds of skills that help in understanding an issue above and beyond just taking in information. So very much I think I still use those skills … even in presentations, keeping people awake.

Community Health Revisited, 1993–1996

By the time Bronwyn's oldest child was in high school, Bronwyn felt ready for full-time work again. Her old position became available in community health in Orange. She applied, and returned to her old job:

> I felt like I was just slipping into an old comfortable shoe again. But with renewed vigour and I think with a lot more experience: life experience and the experience of teaching. I went back into it with a lot more confidence … there was a sense of I did know what I was doing and it was now enhanced with that life experience and extra study that I'd done. And I think, less of a feeling that I had to do it right or that people had to think that I was doing it right. Less expectations I suppose. I had a much more realistic view of what the role was and what I could and couldn't do … 13 years later I knew when I felt out of my depth or I knew what was honest about this relationship. I knew when I could say to this person that I'm not going to fix the situation but we're going to work on it together … I could articulate the realism of the relationship more than I could when I was brand new and trying to make a good impression … And I had a wonderful colleague, a male social worker who had been working there for a couple of years. And he and I got on so well. We still do.

Bronwyn found that working with a male social worker created more opportunities for the service: male clients were encouraged to engage with it and it was now possible to offer joint couple counselling. While she only worked in this job for two and half years, two other projects stand out.

The first was running a group for women who had been in violent relationships:

> one of the highlights of my working career was working with those women … bringing those women together I think was just one of the most powerful things that I had seen in terms of … ending their isolation, helping them to really evaluate where they were at, seeing the relationships in a different light, understanding them, knowing that there were other women in there in that same position. It was almost like I could just sit back and let the work happen there, they were hungry for it.

Strongly encouraged, or *pushed* by Area Social Work Advisor Kate Baxter, Bronwyn presented her first paper on her work with this group to the state Australian Association of Social Workers (AASW) conference held in Bathurst in 1994—"Over the Great Divide". This was the first time an AASW NSW state conference had been held outside Sydney. Kate Baxter was key in organising the conference. Bronwyn recalls: *She would push you to do things and she was very encouraging for us all to represent rural social work and to present a paper.*

The other venture that stands out for Bronwyn was working in a community development project in partnership with community health staff and community members who were consumers. The aim was to get more access and involvement from the community in service delivery. The group developed a newsletter called *MATCH* (More Access To Community Help). On weekends Bronwyn, other staff and community members walked the streets, putting *MATCH* into letterboxes and trying to advocate with other community groups to locate a funding source to print the newsletter:

> And it was a struggle all the time but it was an interesting and meaningful kind of struggle. We weren't just going off on our own ideas about what might work or what the community might want. These were people who we had discovered during the course of our work and offered them a role that was beyond the passive service recipient and they grabbed it, they absolutely grabbed it. And that was just so rewarding. I think seeing that we weren't necessarily in control of that—that was the meaningful part.

One of the people who received the newsletter contacted the group about an anomaly in the disability pension. The *MATCH* group lobbied and were successful in getting the issue resolved. Bronwyn and the group got some funding and wrote and presented a paper together at a big international conference on community health in Sydney. *And that was really something to see these people who had become really fired up about issues.* Finally Bronwyn had had the chance to put her community development skills into practice.

Back to TAFE, 1996–2001

In 1996 Bronwyn and the male colleague with whom she had worked closely followed Kate Baxter back into the Orange campus of TAFE, this time to establish a new community service faculty. At first Bronwyn loved it, bringing her social work values, knowledge and skills together with her education side. She was writing state-wide modules for one of the subjects, and meeting other welfare workers. However, once Kate went further into management, Bronwyn as the next most senior teacher felt impelled to accept an offer to become Acting Head Teacher:

> And so what I found myself immersed in now was timesheets, meetings, budgets, all the things I hated, and hardly any teaching. So it was grievances, it was timetabling teachers, it was, how did I find myself here? I don't want to do this anymore. And I didn't, I didn't enjoy it, I became really unhappy. I felt out of my depth in so many of those meetings because I don't get these things, I don't want to get them, I don't want to be responsible for them. So five-year plans and, that's Kate, she was great at that. It wasn't me. I was good at plonk me in front of a class and, with real people and I could work with that. But I couldn't work with timesheets and timetables and five-year plans, I just couldn't. Didn't like the language. I didn't get it and didn't want to be there.

Escape to London, 2000

With her adult children travelling overseas, Bronwyn decided to fulfil a lifelong dream and go overseas to work herself: *By this stage I was in my mid to late 40s. And once again a supportive husband, who helped me run away from home.*

She took long service leave and within two days of being in England she had a job in East London in child protection, in the Newham Social Services Children in Need Team:

> the work conditions there were so different. You had to take a bus to go to home visits, and I found that incredibly amusing. So even, from my first job in Bathurst where here's your car that you can take home to landing in this job saying oh we can help pay your bus ticket if you bring back the receipt, [laughs] it's like really? And I remember, and we were packed into this, it was an old fire station in Eastham. So thick in the middle of East London, culturally diverse, just amazing. Such a difference to Orange rural community and, in Australia. And was such a great experience.

Bronwyn delighted in the diversity and flexibility of her new workplace, learning about child protection, working with interpreters, thoroughly enjoying her new colleagues. She noted how well respected Australian social workers were, wondering if it was *a bit of grounding in principles of social work ... maybe around ethics and reflective practice.* Being in East London taught her that she wanted to be working with people, not timetabling and timesheets, and she decided to go back into practice. After a great family holiday in Europe Bronwyn *came home to reality and back to TAFE and I was unhappier than ever there.*

A Home in Mental Health, 2001 to Present

After about six months back in TAFE, Bronwyn applied for and moved into a job in mental health—a position that was split between child and adolescent mental health in the community and an inpatient unit at a large regional mental health facility:

> So I applied and got the job and that's how I landed where I am now and this is the longest I have ever been in a job, so this is coming up, I'm in my 14th year now, yeah. So 13 years I've been working in mental health in the same, well the position's changed a little bit but basically still in mental health.

After a few years in the job Bronwyn began to feel uncomfortable and to question the accepted practices. Were they pathologising the adolescents they were counselling? Were they encouraging self-harm and long-term dependence?

The solution to many questions came in the form of systemic family therapy training, provided from Sydney. Bronwyn and one other psychologist *got it*. A systemic family approach meant that fathers were included more—no longer could it be assumed that dads weren't interested. Strategies such as writing letters, being curious, circular questioning—Bronwyn found the impact on families was profound.

Other issues in the team were emerging: lack of purpose, reactive service provision rather than inclusive planning, which led Bronwyn into focusing on a group (this group was run in the inpatient setting) that became a strengths-based group about being a parent with a mental illness. The focus became what's right with me, not what's wrong with me.

Soon Bronwyn found herself being offered to act as allied health manager in the hospital while her own allied health manager was acting in a more senior position:

> and I suddenly started saying why have I done this? Here am I again I've been taken away from working with people on the ground which is what I like, and here am I again doing timesheets. And going to meetings around five-year plans, and I don't want to do this.

So Bronwyn declined the offer to continue as acting allied health manager and went back to her substantive senior social worker position, a position she has held ever since. At last she has found the role that she wants—combining a clinical element and a supervision role. In 2008 she went full time for the hospital, leaving the community team role behind. Having only one team and one site to focus on was a relief.

> That keeps me excited and rewarded and, you know working with the families in this unit that I'm on has just been the best thing out. We've got a great sense of being together and it's taken the staff along with them too which has been really lovely and the executive who now, you know, talk about our open days and our support group for the carers and you know I'm down in Sydney in March presenting to the benchmarking, the state wide benchmarking group about this program and they use it to advertise the services. I don't mind because what I get out of it is those times when we sit down with the families and we have a great laugh and they're saying well let us take that on, we'll do that or we'll do, and the residents seeing families that they haven't seen for 24 years and that's the reward I get. I don't get that sitting in a meeting with the executive [laughing].

Important Contributions and Recognitions

For Bronwyn her important contributions come from her practices with people that create connections, link strengths and, when she can, *sit back and watch the explosions happen.*

> What am I proud of? … I suppose those things that I'd see as achievements involving the answer to my previous question about the connection. So the domestic violence group had that kind of explosion. The MATCH newsletter had that explosion. The carers open day had that explosion. Those sort of things are the ones that stand out, that I feel proud that I had a role in initiating. And … I suppose this is where pride comes in. I think if I wasn't there, they probably wouldn't have happened.

Having clients recognise her contributions through her strengths-based approach, and skilled application of fundamental or core social skills is also one of Bronwyn's contributions. She remembers a woman who thanked her at the end of the intervention for being *the only person who had been able to work with her as a "normal" person.* Another recognition is from a family who had terrible ongoing—and so far still unsolvable—problems with their daughter over many years. *When I left CAMHS the parents gave me a big bunch of flowers and told me that I was the only one who had stuck by them.*

Colleagues have also recognised Bronwyn:

> It was an invitation to a farewell for a psychiatrist who was retiring and who I had worked with when I was in the CAMHS team which I had left five years previously. This particular psychiatrist used to fly up from Sydney once a month (as most of them do) and when he first arrived he announced that he did not like working with psychologists and social workers. However we struck up a good relationship and worked with many families together … So it was with great surprise that I received this invitation to his farewell after so many years since working together. I arrived at Government House expecting a large function, only to find that it was a lunch for just 12 of us with the Governor (Marie Bashir). This made me feel even more privileged. I guess you could say that the barriers he presented when he first came to CAMHS about working with social workers were somehow overcome.

The Current Stage

Currently Bronwyn faces many challenges in her professional life at the large inpatient facility. Following her lifelong pattern, in addition to her full-time job she has continued to study, enrolling in a Doctor of Social Work course to research lived experiences of recovery in an inpatient mental health setting. An important part of her study involves trying to understand and find ways to address the dissonance she observes in everyday practice, between a genuine passion to help and behaviours that contradict this. *I can't make sense of what I see in practice and what I hear and truly believe people really feel.*

Another challenge is how in the new buildings, with electronic surveillance, cutting down of old trees and restricting freedom, the best aspects of "asylum" are being destroyed. At the same time, despite the will to improve care, she and her colleagues are *suddenly finding ourselves in an environment of care delivery that is worse and more restrictive and more custodial, more contained and less conducive to recovering well.*

Nonetheless, Bronwyn has hope and anger on her side, and support from colleagues and the families of consumers. When asked, she says that satisfaction in her work comes from: *connecting people I think. And then sitting back and watch the explosions happen ... How can I connect all that strength stuff together and make something happen? Channel the power of that? Yeah, that's what I enjoy.*

Analysis of Qualities/Character

Drawing on Bronwyn's biographic analysis, the following qualities have been identified. They are not presented in any particular order, nor do they have any logical sequencing.

Achievement Orientation

Bronwyn comes from a family where academic achievement was highly valued and celebrated by her parents. To meet those expectations, Bronwyn focused on doing well in her studies: *I liked being at the top of the class or I liked getting the highest mark in my project*. Except in her university days, the quality of high academic achievement orientation instilled in her early life continued to influence even her adult life. When she received the college medal, first thing she did was to inform her parents. In her further research and higher degree program, Bronwyn has maintained a distinction or high distinction grade. The sense of academic achievement was and is important to her. How has this quality made a difference or played out in her practice?

Love of Learning and Teaching

Closely linked to academic achievement, Bronwyn's biography shows a life-long love of learning, which she traces to her mother and maternal grandfather, a teacher who encouraged everyone to learn. Bronwyn's mother always admired him for his teaching ability and encouraged herself and her children to learn, though her own desire to learn was somewhat thwarted by family life and motherhood. In her 50s, Bronwyn's mother enrolled in a school for seniors and began studying French and philosophy. Her learning spirit continued even in her 90s. In her own life Bronwyn has also cultivated the habit of continuous learning, Her many certificates, degrees and diplomas are testimony to this commitment.

Bronwyn's success in learning shows in her ability to learn quickly and adapt to a range of work contexts, appreciating the common social work themes across them. When discussing her experience in the UK multicultural environment, Bronwyn said:

> I worked with different backgrounds, different approaches and the different people. But it was interesting that the family issues, the emotions and the relationships were just no different to anywhere else … the things that were important were your respect, your genuineness, your ability to listen. All those core skills, it didn't matter what the cultural diversity was, they were going to work for you. And that's what people respond to, no matter what. So I learned that very quickly.

Bronwyn quickly learned about the Child Protection Act, intake work, home visits and paperwork requirements in London. She focused more on similarities than differences, which is a feature of her approach to teaching, another treasured thread in her professional life:

> I really enjoyed that and decided then that maybe teaching would fit more perhaps with the family life at the time, I love … experiential learning … providing those opportunities for people to experience things not me being the all knower … seeing people change and become aware of certain aspects around themselves and the way that they related to others. I really enjoyed that.

Exploring the Links Between Social Work and Teaching

Bronwyn's biography demonstrates her active application of social work to teaching. In regards to one of her teaching assignments, Bronwyn had this to say:

> this was the ideal job, I love teaching, and yet I've really loved social work and here am I now being able to do both in the development of these courses in the teaching of these skills, and at the same time I was learning because if I'm teaching about social processes or social justice or whatever I have to know what I'm talking about. So it made me really be up to date with what was going on, or pretty much up to date. And the excitement of talking students into a new way of thinking about the world, and it was lovely; I really enjoyed those times.

When teaching at TAFE, Bronwyn appreciated the links between the interpersonal and relationship skills she had learned in social work, and also the group work skills:

> Relationships are central to so many things and particularly social work because it is about knowing the person across from you, it's about understanding and having that empathy, really tuning in with them, being with them, and I don't think that's any different in teaching either.
>
> And I think the group work skills that I got, and I did major in group work at university, they were particularly the skills that I used in an educational sense. I still think they're just as important in an educational sense as they are in the social work sense.

Early Sensitivity to the Needs of Others

One of Bronwyn's earliest memories of being aware of the needs of others was her response to the plight of the boys from the Salvation Army Boys' Home who attended her primary school. She attributes this early sensitivity to her mother: *It was actually my mother's idea to invite the boys to my birthday party. I attribute my sensitivity to other people's needs to this action of my mother's.* Later, while studying social work and influenced by the Whitlam era, this sensitivity blossomed into Bronwyn's dream of *working with oppressed communities and helping them move out of the oppression.*

Feminism

Examining the ideas and arguments of feminism, and understanding it as an emerging movement in the 1970s, inspired Bronwyn and opened a new world for her. She discussed the shifts at personal and professional levels this caused. She said: *It shifted me from all those values that my parents had raised me within to this whole different ... way of thinking about the world that's not defined in this masculine kind of way.*

Influences of feminism were really personal to Bronwyn and she appreciated the link between the personal and the political. Later she threw herself into motherhood and at the same time nurtured in her own daughters the ability/quality to question the existing world order from the perspective of feminism.

The Art of Listening

Like the ideas of feminism, another factor that inspired Bronwyn in her social work course was the art of listening. Deeply embedded in this is valuing and respecting people. In the social work course and beginning practice, she realised how difficult it was to listen and how crucial it was to *discover the difference between wanting to fix and allowing a solution to emerge through listening.*

Such a realisation has helped Bronwyn practise with a difference—not only with people she works with, but also in her research. Her selection of a phenomenological *deep listening* methodology and her passionate commitment to recovery principles and social work's potential for leadership in recovery practice, reflects her deep respect for the deceptively simple tool of listening. Over the years, careful listening has become one of her traits and priorities: *I see the most powerful changes from those very basic skills.*

An important note is that careful listening does not preclude preparation. Bronwyn believes in preparing well for any tasks or role. Whether it is interviewing clients or their families, appearing for an interview or examination, good preparation is necessary.

Relationships and Team Work—Working with, not for

Relationships are fundamental to Bronwyn's personal and professional life. Her life story revealed how she values a small number of close, long-term friends, some from her earliest school days. Looking back on her school days, she says, *a feature of my life that has influenced my decision to go into social work and probably sustained me there is about relationships.*

Bronwyn also developed personal relationships with work colleagues; for example, her male colleague who is still a close friend after many years.

In discussing her professional life, Bronwyn frequently refers to the term *team*. It may be appreciating the team (*we had a great team of people; nice team*), forming and developing the team (*we formed a really good team; allowed me to really see the team grow*), recognising the role of purpose in team building (*we're all in it together, we're all going to help; the purpose of community health was uniting*), or it may be the team spirit (*there was a camaraderie there; we were all supportive of each other; there was a really strong sense of team*). These phrases suggest that Bronwyn recognises and appreciates the importance of the teamwork in practice; she likes to work as a member of the team or lead it. These are highly valued qualities in social work practice.

Working with People, not with Paper—Choosing Clinical Work Over Management Roles

Linked to her commitment to foundational social work is Bronwyn's insistence that she wants to work with people, not with paper. She refuses to work with timesheets, timetables and five-year plans. Bronwyn said, *I am happy to sit at the bottom of the ladder and work with real people, that's all I wanted to do. Because that keeps me grounded and keeps me linked to a people world, rather than a paper world.*

Bronwyn has been fighting *to return to basics as a grade one social worker* in an inpatient unit in a mental health facility. Her first priority is to see people as persons, not problems; and even if changes do not occur in the short term, to remain there—to listen and connect with human beings for the long term. Bronwyn loves clinical work. Working with families keeps her excited and rewarded. She believes that *the most powerful changes come from those very basic skills … In my time I've had to fight to go back to basics, fight, fight, fight.* She said:

> Yeah, often there is the pressure to move up. Now I think some of that initially was because I was one of few people in a very small pond … but as it's gone on I think maybe I can articulate things well and they think oh she'd be a good spokesperson … or maybe there's an assumption that it's a logical progression always ever upwards in your career and that I'm at a stage where I'd like to be on top and be the top manager. I've never ever wanted, never ever sought that out. So it's been a struggle in some ways because I've had to say no and I haven't said no in the past because I think I'm … cheating myself out of this or there's a responsibility to the family because this comes with more money and I could be earning more money for the family coffers, all those other kind of external things when inside I knew I didn't want this.

At the very beginning, when Bronwyn became a team leader at the end of her first year of practice, she wondered how she was chosen for such a role. As a health social worker, her small stint at the social security department left her feeling very different from social workers in administrative roles, despite their ability to change lives. In TAFE she hated being an Acting Head Teacher. In health she strongly questioned the Allied Health Manager role after she had accepted it. *I was acting Allied Health Manager and I suddenly started saying why have I done this ... here am I again doing timesheets. And going to meetings around five-year plans, and I don't want to do this, this is why I got out of TAFE.*

After the recent merger in her regional mental health service, the position of Head of Social Work was created and Bronwyn was one of the most likely people to be appointed. Reflecting on her three management experiences, this fourth time Bronwyn consciously declined the opportunity. She said:

> I knew if I put my head to it I could do it but I didn't like it and that soon got in the way of my doing it well I think. It didn't sit well with my need to do something well, and if I can't do it well then I don't want to do it and I think that's what finally got in the way.

Bronwyn had decided that management was not for her:

> I would be in some sort of leadership role perhaps and that's what flattered me in the past, these offers to do that, so I said of course I can lead that, of course I can do that, but it didn't bring me any happiness [laughing]. So I guess it was realising all of those things and … I think I had to let go of expectations, my own expectations and perhaps other people's expectations of me; I had to let go of that and say no.

Questioning

Questioning is a key theme in Bronwyn's biography. First, she began vehemently questioning "stay-at-home mother" traditional values and, as her life developed, she questioned whether she had ended up following the same traditional values she had initially rejected. Within the mental health setting, Bronwyn began questioning whether the prevailing practice approach was pathologising children and also questioned the assumption that "father is not interested". It was a revelation for Bronwyn to see how circular questioning helped families to gain further insight. She said, *I started to question again why, what I was doing and whether or not it was really working for the clientele.* Such questioning extended to teams, management and organisations. Raising questions and thinking about them is a useful habit and a foundational step towards reflective practice.

Managing Different Values?

We have discussed how Bronwyn quietly rejected her parents' espoused values, yet acknowledged the irony that: *Much as we rejected our parents' values ... we found ourselves falling very much into a traditional lifestyle of marriage and children.*

Apparently she was not always as quiet as she thought she was about traditional family values, noting how apparent contradictions continue through the generations:

> I remember absolutely shocking my mother when I rang her to announce I was pregnant because she never thought I would have a baby … I must have been quite vocal … rejecting all those traditional things that women were expected to do … and here I was pregnant within the first year of our marriage … Looking back it's really interesting to see just how much of the traditional pattern I ended up pursuing. A mortgage before 30, three children before 30, married before 30, and I look at my children now and I think what's wrong with you? … Did I push the feminist line too hard? I just want to be a grandma now, come on! … But you know it's so different now. They really have kind of rejected those, the automatic values I suppose that I thought I had rejected and then ended up living out … though I find it really interesting these days girls who get married change their name instantly, they don't even think about it.

Work/Family Conflicting Balance—Gender Issue

Throughout her life Bronwyn has dealt with competing expectations of learning, academic achievements and having a professional career on one hand, and getting married and raising a family on the other. She attributes these mixed messages to her mother, who encouraged her children to learn a lot and also have a family life. Bronwyn managed to take on a series of part-time positions and formal study throughout the 13 years when her children were young. She is clear that her husband's support has been vital in helping her to manage these conflicting gender-role demands. Despite such co-operation and support, with her acute awareness of feminism, Bronwyn questions whether she has drifted between the conflicting expectations rather than actively managing them: *I often feel that with my life things would just present themselves and I would go, oh, okay. That'll do. Instead of me having this driving passion to be somewhere in the world, I'd just go alright, that looks ok.*

Awareness of Boundary and Role Issues

While raising young children when she was home, Bronwyn assisted her husband in his newsagency business by working behind the counter. When she resumed the full-time social work job in community health, she was adamant about ceasing the newsagency work, though it was an important business for her husband. This conscious decision in the face of pressure to support the family venture demonstrates Bronwyn's awareness of the ethical dimensions surrounding boundary and role complexities in rural communities.

Pushing to Do More—Hard Work for Learning and Hard Work with People

Bronwyn has pushed herself and worked hard most of her life. For example, while raising young children, she pushed herself to do the diploma of primary education, thoroughly enjoying how the experiences of her children growing fed directly into the course content, notwithstanding the tough study regime very late at night described in her biography, which she combined with part-time teaching and family life.

Motherhood and part-time work were not enough for Bronwyn. She said, *I wanted something more than the motherhood and the casual work scene. I wanted to further myself a bit more and take this opportunity and that's when I went back to study and got my Dip. Ed.*

She remembered how an advisor was very good in encouraging and pushing colleagues, including Bronwyn, to do more, and that is what Bronwyn does as a senior social work practitioner:

> I am always pushing them to do things that are beyond their comfort zone because I think that was really good, that's what I really respected with an advisor, and is what probably got me to just step that little bit further and test myself out a bit more and probably be more effective in that way because I was being a little more rigorous about what I was doing or had more commitment or accountability. And that's what I tried to do with my social work team too because I can see their potential, I can see where they're shining.

The example about working with consumers to produce the *MATCH* newsletter also shows how Bronwyn struggled and worked hard to achieve her ideals of working with rather than for people. Throughout her interview Bronwyn emphasises this theme of learning to work with, not for, people. While working with families, when members see a new understanding of each other and feel capable of doing something with each other, Bronwyn feels rewarded. She equally feels rewarded when responsibility is shared rather than left to a social worker alone to fix it. She noted that with increasing confidence she was more able to work with, rather than for, others. For her this is a quality or ability that comes with experience and hard work.

Supervision—Receiving and Offering

Regular professional supervision is crucial both from personal and practice perspectives, more so in rural areas where it is difficult to access. Bronwyn's practice shows how she was receptive to supervision and as a senior social worker how she offered supervision to other social workers. She recalled as a beginning social worker having group supervision sessions offered by two senior social workers who were periodically flown from Sydney to Bathurst:

> They were wonderful, and it was such a breath of fresh air. It was a wonderful opportunity to have that group supervision and they, my memory of them is just such mature and experienced people, something that we desperately needed out here … because there were

> very few of us who weren't new grads. And those of us who weren't only had a few years' experience behind them. Such support in rural communities was incredibly important for us … as it connected to a broader, wider system.

When Bronwyn worked in the child and mental health area, she appreciated the regular supervision and training in family therapy offered from Sydney. Later, as a senior social worker in the hospital, she was responsible for the provision of supervision, which she loved: *I always enjoyed provision of supervision, as well as receiving supervision.*

Focus on Opportunities for Change

In her practice, Bronwyn focuses on opportunities for change, which she found at the inpatient mental health facility. Bronwyn is *interested in making the hospital experience for people a better one.* She adds: *I think I just had a clearer view of what could be done there. So that's why I became a full-time social worker at the hospital inpatient setting.*

She saw the opportunities for long-term change:

> But I think I'm very fortunate in the long-stay units that I've got that time to get to know these people that when, you know their loved ones at this stage aren't going anywhere in a hurry so we've got time to build a relationship, we've got time to build trust, we've got time to really work with them about any decisions around what concerns their loved one.

Bronwyn's *explosions*, forming groups, the *MATCH* newsletter and carers open day show her passion for change. Working outside the expected norms (for example, careerist), she has demonstrated silent activism and initiated change in the immediate milieu.

Gaining Confidence: "Can I Do It?" to "I Can Do It"

During her student days and placement at councils, Bronwyn was inspired by the Australian Assistance Plan and in her ideal world she wanted to work for communities to change them. But at that time Bronwyn thought that that kind of work *may be a little beyond her capabilities*. She said:

> I don't think I had the confidence to be out there publicly. Like at that stage that whole community development was about being like a political activist and being out there and I just didn't see I had that confidence or that conviction about a cause that would give me the confidence to be out there and lead any kind of political activist kind of role.

Although Bronwyn fancied community work, she felt more confident about work with individuals and small groups. She said:

> I knew in the end that I'm more a one on one person or a small group person or a, yeah working with people individually rather than on mass. Yeah so it was maybe a sense of comfort or discomfort around the skills required. [pause] Maybe a, yeah maybe it was more that I didn't trust that I would understand the cause enough to be out there upfront.

When Bronwyn assumed her first social work position, her confidence appears to have been at a different level. She recollected, *I was pretending I knew what I was doing when I was maybe panicking a bit inside saying am I doing this right, is this okay, I don't know, where do I go from here.*

Yet she became a team leader at the end of her first year but after a few years marriage, children and family took priority over career. Over a period of 13 years, along with raising a young family, Bronwyn took several part-time positions in social work and teaching at TAFE and acquiring formal qualifications. Following the 13 years of juggling between young family and part-time study and work, when she joined as full-time social worker in community health, her level of confidence was high.

Bronwyn gradually built her confidence into practice. It appears that during the beginning of her career inside herself she raised the question *Can I do it?* though outside she hid that question and did her best. Later in life, work and study experiences significantly enhanced her confidence to the level of *I can do it.*

Sense of Frustration and Helplessness and Resistance to Managerialism

Having carefully observed over the years the management changes and approaches, both as an insider and outsider, Bronwyn's narration suggests a sense of frustration and helplessness, and to some extent resistance to managerialism. She finds the *environment of care delivery worse and more restrictive and more custodial, and more contained, and less conducive to recovering well.* It appears that corporate and management approaches are suffocating the ethos of social work practice. Bronwyn observes:

> Somehow that message comes through all the time, and you kind of give up after a while, because you're fighting, fighting, fighting for one little room or something. And then you lose the picture of the whole service and what it's doing, because it's all progressed so far that there's no going back on it and they have their blueprints of what a unit needs to look like within a certain budget.
>
> When I first went, there was a more humanistic approach to inpatient care, it has actually become less humanistic over the years with the advent of these new buildings with all these risk-management and security-conscious processes that are in place.

As the managerial trend is pervasive in all spheres, what kind of impact will it have on the qualities and character of social workers?

Commitment, Passion and Hope

The sense of frustration and helplessness notwithstanding, Bronwyn through her research and practice experience has found commitment, passion and hope in the current mental health setting, where she has been working for the last 14 years:

There's still a lot of hope that we can hang onto, and turn this into something that is much more valuable for people with an illness.

I was quite gobsmacked at their [staff] level of passion and commitment to this area of work, and the number of people that have been hooked by mental health, and I think I'm probably one of them too … but the core connection I think is this humanistic outlook, this understanding of people in a situation that's out of their control and the empathy that comes with that and the understanding and wanting to understand and help them through that—that seems to be this core component of passion that people feel.

I suppose the difference with mental health is I've always had those doubts, but maybe I'm just more optimistic that there's a way through them or something, I don't know. [pause] And why mental health would grab me in that way I don't really know either, maybe it's just such a mystery of the mind that keeps you fascinated, and confronts you with different ways of looking at the world that it is confronting but I think it's very good for you too to view things in very different ways. And people who have those challenges on a daily basis force you, not deliberately, but you know if you really tune in you do see the world in a very different way.

Conclusion

The life story of a rural-based social work practitioner, Bronwyn Hyde, offers many lessons and insights for a careful reader. From a tentative start, *I didn't have any strong urge or passionate interest or anything, I just knew I had to do something*, Bronwyn's practice story has not turned out to be just 'something". With her priority of grassroots-level people and colleagues, Bronwyn has made significant contributions in rural/regional areas and beyond, particularly in mental health. Wending her way through social work and education, grounded in feminism, lifelong learning, family and close relationships, Bronwyn's story reveals the importance of social work's foundational elements: respect, listening, relationships and the quest for social justice. Her idea of creating connections, linking strengths so that people's own power creates an *explosion*, is one of the gifts from her story.

Chapter 8
I Cannot Give up, I Cannot Give up on the Children—Bernadette McMenamin, AO

Manohar Pawar and Linda Briskman

Bernadette McMenamin's biography presents an exceptional life story and list of professional accomplishments. Overcoming early adversities in life, Bernadette completed social work education, began her social work practice career in public housing, vehemently fought for social justice and became a leading campaigner against child sex abuse. Bernadette founded Child Wise™ Limited, a child protection charity with a local and global mission, based in Melbourne, Australia, and she was Chief Executive Officer for more than 22 years.

As the National Director of Child Wise, Bernadette was responsible for developing innovative child abuse prevention programs and campaigns, nationally and internationally. Of particular note is the enactment of the Child Sex Tourism law in 1994 to make sex with children overseas a prosecutable offence in Australia, and her advocacy for its implementation. In recognition of these sustained efforts and achievements Child Wise received a number of awards. In 2004 Bernadette was the Victorian finalist for Australian of the Year and was awarded the Order of Australia (AO) in June of that year. In 2005, she won the Entrepreneur of the Year award in the Social Entrepreneur category for the Southern Region of Australia and in 2006 she was a Victorian finalist in the Telstra Business Women's Award. The analysis of her life story and professional practice offers inspiring lessons and qualities.

M. Pawar (✉)
Charles Sturt University, Wagga Wagga, Australia
e-mail: mpawar@csu.edu.au

L. Briskman
Western Sydney University, Sydney, Australia
e-mail: l.briskman@westernsydney.edu.au

M. Pawar et al. (eds.), *Empowering Social Workers*,
DOI 10.1007/978-981-10-3809-9_8

Early Life

Bernadette Mary McMenamin was born in 1958, in Birmingham, England, and was raised in extremely difficult circumstances by her Irish parents, who themselves were deprived of love and support when they were young. Her maternal grandmother died when her mother was four and her maternal grandfather passed away in Ireland when her mother was seven. Bernadette's mother looked after her two younger siblings and they died of dysentery; the older siblings went to the city to work. *The food was very scarce and they had to go to the beach and eat seaweed.* Bernadette's father left home when he was ten, as his father had died and his mother had remarried.

Bernadette's parents were *very uneducated, but very sharp/street wise*. They had very "black and white"/racist views about the world and did not appreciate the black people's presence in their neighbourhood in England, where a lot of Caribbean or Jamaican people resided. The neighbourhood also became an Irish hub. Whereas Bernadette wondered, *what's wrong with black people, what's wrong with their music, what's wrong with all the people that my father spoke about*? Bernadette said, *from a very early age I believe that I had a social conscience*. Her childhood and adolescent years were replete with neglect, different forms of abuse and traumatic experiences. *I think five years of age I was kissing a black boy, you know, just [kissing sound] an innocent little kiss up the lane, and my mother found me and I was spanked until my bottom was raw.*

At the age of six, Bernadette experienced sexual abuse, but was frightened to tell her parents (Lunn 2012). They were alcoholics and knew disciplining children only through physical punishment and perhaps that is how they were brought up. Bernadette reflected: *We were all beaten, not with hands, but with sticks, straps ... the domestic violence we used to see in our home was horrific.*

When Bernadette was 12 years old, her parents moved from England to Australia and they settled in St Kilda, Melbourne. Bernadette was the youngest in the family, with an older brother and sister, and most of the time the children were on their own. To Bernadette it was not a loving home. When she tried to hug her, her mother would always freeze up. Such a response raised questions in Bernadette's mind. Her parents were *a very tight-knit couple*. Bernadette depicted the neglect experienced in her childhood:

> We were home alone a lot, and we didn't get a lot of affection, physical affection. We didn't get what we wanted to; we got what our parents wanted us to have and that was that ... But in terms of physical affection there was none. It was very hard. They, you know, they wouldn't, it wasn't like they would, they were always too busy, always too busy for us. I mean they were trying to make the world a better place for their children, and in their minds the harder they worked the better their children would be, and they didn't understand that children need love and care and compassion. I can't even remember hugging my mother. I can't remember hugging my father.

Hugs were replaced with drugs. Bernadette was exposed to drugs when she was 13, when she used heroine for the first time. She became sexually active and associated with *juvenile delinquents*. One day, a response to a knock on the door resulted in her father's best friend trying to rape her and he fled when her friends, who were there for a sleepover, ran out of her bedroom after hearing screams. When her father returned from work, Bernadette said:

> I told my father, I marched up to him and he just didn't say anything to me, he just looked at me and didn't respond, and continued his friendship with this, his friend up until he died. And that, that was shattering because I had to see this person …
>
> Never sitting down and talking to you, and that's when awful things that did happen to me, and I was pretty, you know, gutsy, I would tell them and they would just say, "I don't want to know, I don't want to know. I don't want to know because I'm sure at the end of the day you were somehow responsible for it." I got earrings and my father called me a whore, you know, things like that. It was, at the same time I loved them and that's what makes me feel, like I've worked with so many children and so many families, and no matter how hard it is for some children they still want to be with their mum and dad. I mean I ran away a dozen times but always came back …
>
> I was a pretty out of control teenager. I mean it, it stands, I mean you know, they set certain boundaries and my reaction was to break those boundaries. I'd disappear for two days and come home and then I'd get a flogging, and that wouldn't do a great deal. That would be the next time. So yes, I think it certainly wasn't in my teens that I realised that in their own way that they did love us.

When Bernadette was 15 she was caught in a devastating situation when she was walking home during the night time. She narrates:

> I was gang raped and thrown out of a car in the middle of the bush in the middle of nowhere, and fortunately a truck driver found me, brought me to the police. The police blamed me for being in the wrong place at the wrong time, and drove me home. I had cracked ribs, I was pretty beaten up, my face was like a bent mushroom, but it was just something that I couldn't tell anyone. So after, I tried to talk to my parents about this and they, well my mother just didn't want to know, she didn't want to hear, she didn't, you know, like if anything went wrong it was my fault, I'd done something wrong. So she didn't want to hear it. My friends didn't want to talk about it so I was sort of left alone with this staggering feeling of doom and gloom and sadness. Therapy wasn't something that was around at the time and I'd never really thought about it because I was quite young, I was 15. But I became very angry, I became very angry and very paranoid for a while, and you know, sleeping with knives under my mattress and hammers under my bed, and I was frightened.

To leave this traumatic experience behind, Bernadette travelled to the UK, stayed at her uncle's home for a few weeks and was on her own for more than a year. She undertook menial jobs in offices and pubs, living with the deep thoughts of what had happened and what was happening to her. After returning to Australia, she went back to school and studied anthropology, sociology and legal studies as she developed a passion for learning more. To dim the deep pain she also turned to drugs, as they were easily accessible in St Kilda and she was off and on drugs for about seven years. To pay for drugs she became a sex worker and was caught up in a vicious circle of drug dealers and criminals, who exploited her. At school, encouragement and praise from teachers helped her. They encouraged Bernadette to question everything. From this she was motivated to study more, and she did well in the Higher School Certificate. Alongside sex work and drug addiction, she enrolled in humanities at Monash University.

Bernadette experienced a life-threatening situation involving drug gangsters. To completely disassociate from such characters she decided to move away from them, although *it was not that easy*, and she went to Adelaide to study at Flinders University. It was a turning point for Bernadette. She enrolled in a double major in sociology and politics and she wanted to change the world. At the end of her study, when she faced the question of what to do next, *honours or what*, she consulted a careers counsellor, who suggested that she consider becoming a social worker. At that time Bernadette's response and understanding of social work was:

> Oh, social worker? Aren't they the baddies? Aren't they the people that wear, you know, those pearl jumpers and take children off people? I mean that was my knowledge of social work. And she said, "No, look, there's just so many options that you can do, that you can take …" I thought, "Well, I might as well give it a go".

Social Work Education and Training

Bernadette returned to Melbourne and enrolled in the social work course at La Trobe University. A few years away from Melbourne had helped her *break old relationships*. When she looked at social work subjects and the social change focus in it, Bernadette said, *I naturally gravitated to it*. While doing the course, two crucial turning points were concepts of politicisation and empowerment. On Orientation Day, she *chose to join the Marijuana Reform Party, wanted to be a rebel and stand up against convention*. She got herself onto the student council and found her voice. The social work course helped her to argue, to discuss, to analyse and to question. Her recollections of studying social work were as follows:

> for the first time in my life I felt like I was good at something, you know, I could actually see myself in this helping other people, and I have no doubt that my empathy came from my own wounds, not that I lived out my abuse or neglect through other people; that was definitely something I never did. It just gave me a heightened sense of compassion I think. So after social work, throughout social work the things that really appealed to me were radical social work—that we could change the world and that the rules for radicals and all of those people organised, they can bring about change. That really resonated with me because I think I felt so disempowered in my younger years that to find a way to empower myself was a godsend, it really was.

During the course, Bernadette hated her mental health fieldwork placement, as she thought it was *horrible and awful*. In mental health, *she could not see light through the tunnel*. She observed *a very repressive system filled with drugs*, which is why she did not wish to work in that field.

Her next fieldwork placement, public housing in West Heidelberg, provided an opportunity for her to *organise tenants on the housing estate to help to empower them, to take more ownership and more pride and more responsibility around their community*. Bernadette was pleased to receive extremely positive feedback in the

Bachelor of Social Work (BSW) course. She received an A grade for everything and graduated with distinction, which enhanced her confidence.

First Social Worker Job

Her placement at the public housing in West Heidelberg led to a first social worker job at the same agency. Bernadette continued to work with residents to identify and address their needs and issues. Her role involved preparing a report and training residents for interviews. She prepared a report that was launched by a government minister, and this resulted in allocation of funds to improve the estate. In her first job, Bernadette recollected what she had learned and how it helped her to gain confidence:

> I learned how to use the media, I learned how to sort of mobilise people, learned how to write a report with recommendations, so yes, you can do it. So that was, that to me was an omen that, that I was on the right track, that I could really make a difference and help make a difference to people's lives.

Second Job: Manager/Community Development Officer, Flemington Tenants Association

Building on her experience in West Heidelberg, Bernadette embraced the challenges at one of the most notorious public housing estates in Flemington. She spoke of her passion for community development and activist activities. People were scared to go into the Flemington public housing estate both day and night. Bernadette worked with another social worker to gain significant improvements by engaging residents. Bernadette said:

> We had an open door policy, we dealt with everything that came through that door whether it be child abuse, whether it be domestic violence, whether it be needing some money or you know, some food, whether it was a feud with their neighbours, whether it was a need for another house; everything, everything came through that door. And you know, it really kept you on your toes to assist people.

Major achievements included physical improvements to housing and lighting; establishment of the first multicultural security service; provision of community gardens and murals; and an improved sense of safety among residents—and a reduction in vandalism. Additionally, several ethnic groups formed, as well as a number of different committees. Bernadette described it as *we lived in Utopia*. Activism included rent strikes, petitions and blocking of a road on Melbourne Cup Day. This was to lobby for the installation of traffic lights near the estate for the safety of both children and adults. Bernadette was proud of her achievements over a period of nearly ten years in the housing estate and found it difficult to leave the job.

During her holidays, she visited Bangkok, Cambodia and Bali and fell in love with those countries to such an extent that she actively sought an overseas job.

Despite her lengthy community development experience, it was difficult to obtain a position in international agencies and she found the INGOs (International Non-government Organisations) that she approached to be a closed circle. To fulfil her goal, she began studying international social work by enrolling in the Master of Social Work Course at La Trobe University. While studying she registered her name with Australian Volunteers International (AVI), which first offered an opportunity in the Pacific to work on gender issues, but Bernadette declined as it did not interest her. More than a year later, when the AVI made an offer to set up a campaign in Thailand, Bernadette pounced on it, as she liked campaigning and advocating for people, though at that time as a tenant worker she did not know much about child trafficking and trading. But she had noted the prevalence of child sex abuse during her visits overseas.

Campaigner in Bangkok

With only six weeks notice to take up the AVI position in Bangkok, Bernadette experienced sadness about leaving the housing estate. But the overseas opportunity was too good to pass up. The main role assigned to Bernadette was to build an international network of organisations that had a single vision: to End Child Prostitution, Pornography and Trafficking (ECPAT). She recollected: *There were three of us in a room in the middle of nowhere in Bangkok, and it was my job to identify people in different countries, the USA, the UK, throughout Europe, and try and build a network.*

Bernadette conducted herself professionally and produced positive responses from several countries. She convinced the media to cover the story. As one of the founding members, she effectively assisted in establishing ECPAT's international campaign. However, result-oriented work notwithstanding, Bernadette was not able to appreciate certain aspects of her boss and, due to professional and/or cross-cultural factors, there were differences relating to the working/delegation style between them. After working abroad for around 18 months, Bernadette decided to return to Australia, with a fascinating assignment in hand. Having noted her potential and passion for the issue, the founders of the network appointed her as Executive Officer, gave her $3000 and asked to her to set up a campaign for ECPAT in Australia.

Chief Executive Officer, Child Wise, Formerly ECPAT Australia

Bernadette spearheaded the ECPAT Australia campaign from its inception in 1993 and it is now known as Child Wise, operating in 15 countries. Initially, to set up the wing of ECPAT in Australia, the Uniting Church gave Bernadette a desk, a telephone and a bookcase. With limited resources, it was challenging to set up an organisation, but Bernadette began talking about the issue at various forums. Awareness raising and issue making both occurred through a core question: *Do you know that children overseas are being sexually abused by Australians who travel over there, and they get away with it*? Persistently she raised and discussed the issue until people began listening. She also incorporated ECPAT Australia as an entity with a board of directors. During the initial three or four years, Bernadette did not have any paid job. While building the organisation, as funding was a major issue, she worked at nights as a waitress and days and weekends for the organisation and its campaigning.

The size of public meeting venues increased from small church halls to amphitheatres, where hundreds of people attended. She wrote thousands of letters. To Bernadette, equally important was that she got the media on her side very early: *A media story was called "The Ugly Australians" and it was on the front page of just about every Saturday newspaper, and that really exploded the whole issue Australia-wide*.

Bernadette had also worked on the answer to the issue through legislative reform, education, training and awareness. She campaigned and mobilised people at all levels, including politicians, asking them to support the legislative strategy to address the issue. Bernadette said: *I was up at Parliament all the time, I'd be knocking them down and I'd be banging on the tables and you know, I wouldn't leave until I had an answer*. Bernadette worked closely with politicians of all parties as well as encouraging individuals and agencies to form a campaign. Fund raising was also an important strategy to support the campaign. Most importantly, Bernadette believed in herself and she was optimistic about bringing change.

Her determination and single-minded effort resulted in the successful enactment in Australia of the *Crimes (Child Sex Tourism) Amendment Act 1994*. In subsequent years, other innovative outcomes included lobbying for the tighter immigration regulations for unaccompanied minors, child-friendly legal procedures for child witnesses in child sex tourism cases, a specialised Australian Federal Police team to enforce the Child Sex Tourism law and the Sex Slavery law, and a police hotline for people to report child sex tourism crimes. Several innovative national education campaigns to prevent child sex tourism also have been launched. The Child Wise Tourism program has been implemented in nine South Asian countries to prevent child sex tourism and has been recognised as a model of international best practice. Several innovative education and training programs were designed and offered to prevent and deal with child abuse.

As Chief Executive Officer, Bernadette provided exceptionally committed leadership to overseeing the growth and expansion of Child Wise, which not only worked on campaigning and advocacy, but also developed several benchmarking programs that included high standard education and training materials, and counselling and support. The organisation grew from one person to 14 staff members. In addition, several volunteers supported the organisation. Bernadette reduced her salary and lent the organisation $200,000—which she did not get back—to keep the staff going. She provided opportunities for all staff members to grow, although she admitted: *I was not a great people manager*. She also has helped to establish Child Wise Cambodia. In her three-decade career, Bernadette played a key role in establishing four sustainable organisations, including at public housing estates and initiating change locally, nationally and internationally.

In 2013, Bernadette decided to leave Child Wise, as she was "burnt out" and her organisation was more corporatised, introducing more managerial interventions with which she had significant differences. She had mixed feelings about leaving:

> It's been a long, long time you know, 30 years of advocacy, 23 years of working with Child Wise, always getting up in the morning and having something to be passionate about, always being driven by the fact that every day makes a difference. And there's no doubt that leaving Child Wise has been confusing for me because that's who I am …

Bernadette was *proud of her resilience to stick it out for so long with the odds so hard*. She recounts her time at Child Wise as *glorious times*. She is proud of all she did in her 30-year social work career, which she calls *instinctive*. She was able to create a movement as well as raise a son alone. *So I'm proud of him*. About her programs—Choose with Care, Speaking for Themselves, Child Wise Tourism—she said: *I'm proud of our innovation, I'm proud of my innovation*. She was proud of giving opportunities to people to break into their careers.

Bernadette's ground-breaking work attracted a number of honours and awards. A few notable ones include Officer in the Order of Australia (AO) 2004, for service to the community, particularly through the development of programs in Australia and overseas designed to enhance the rights of children and to protect them from exploitation and abuse; Australian of the Year for Victoria (2004); and Human Rights Award (1996). At the age of 56 at the time of her interview, and now out of Child Wise, Bernadette is quietly contemplating what to do next. Her resolution seems to be: *I cannot give up, I cannot give up on the children ... I will give it everything I have got …I want to give back to the world ...*

Analysis of Qualities/Character

Social Justice at the Core

Constant reference was made by Bernadette to notions of justice. This was clear throughout her entire life. To some extent she illustrates the maxim that "the personal is political". As her biography shows, she experienced hardship during her childhood and young adult life, which created personal insights into injustice and its impact. But she did not just focus on self, as she also witnessed the suffering of others. The binary between the personal and the witnessing across the lifespan wove together in influencing her social justice stance. For example, she referred to being outraged at apartheid injustice when she visited South Africa as a child with her parents. Another early external life influence was growing up in St Kilda, where she observed people needing help. She would provide assistance if she could.

Social justice was not just a belief or ideology for Bernadette, but was put into action. Although not always (in texts) referred to within a social justice paradigm, her belief in people's capabilities was frequently at the centre of her activities. One example of this was her work in Cambodia, where she focused on building local organisations rather than working in a way that made people dependent on the West. In this way, community development principles seem to be at the heart of her endeavours. She worked from the notion that people on the ground have the necessary knowledge. And she worked from the ground to reinforce this. She learned along the way about how to deal with injustice.

Her social justice work was apparent in her motivations for becoming a social worker. Rather than entering the profession with a micro lens, she had a desire to change the world.

The emotional side of social justice was also at the core. She has a big heart, she told us. She said that social workers need warmth and understanding and she is critical of some social workers who she sees as mediocre. She recognises, however, that sustainable change is difficult.

Roots of Activism

Bernadette is proud of her activist activities and the changes she brought about. She is able to stand back and reflect on how her passion for causes came about, although it is not possible to identify one major influence. Some of her empathy, she argues, comes from her own wounds. She recalls how her own abuse was ignored, and this is one motivating factor for her to work to make a difference. This transfers into basic actions such as listening to suffering people and transmitting power to disadvantaged groups.

Some of the influences on her thinking and later action are outlined in the social justice section above. Yet it also seems that as a feisty and questioning child, teenager and adult, it was important to her to overcome stereotypes. This started with the racism that she observed in her own parents.

There was also direct contact with people who inspired her. She attributes much of this to a teacher at her school who encouraged her to question. Then there were her social work educators and education, which became the drivers for her analytical skills. And there were also some social workers who were sources of inspiration. One was Wendy Weeks.[1]

Activism in the workplace was conceived as a gradual progression for Bernadette, evident through her work, particularly her activism on a housing estate where she worked collectively with others to respond to injustice while simultaneously developing skills to take her further along the activist path.

[1]Wendy Weeks was a feminist and activist social worker who, up until her death in 2004, inspired generations of social workers.

She came to work in child sex tourism through serendipity and chance. Although this field chose her, she knew it was where she wanted to be as she was quite sure where she did not want to work—mental health. Never swerving from her belief that child sex tourism was a human wrong that needed to be eliminated, she had what some may see as paradoxical views when it came to perpetrators. Bernadette had some compassion for perpetrators too, and her view related to this is presented under "Empathy across boundaries".

Having strong beliefs resulted in firm and decisive action such as building an organisation that dealt with child sex tourism. Alongside this she applied herself to speaking out, including in the media. Eventually the intersection of belief and action was acknowledged through media recognition and the receipt of awards. But she does not rest on her laurels, recognising that there is still much to be done to achieve the social justice goals to which she aspires. In this way the roots of activism have grown incrementally as an ongoing process.

Personal Attributes: Doggedness and Determination

Although stating that she has a big heart, she has learned, perhaps along the way, to invoke the hard side of herself to make a point. In so doing she is not too fussed about whether she fits in or not, particularly when, as CEO of an organisation, she avoided what was expected, such as cocktail parties and small talk.

She admits that some of this was due to shyness, but also a realisation that people do not warm to being told about the "nasty" side of life, such as children with syphilis. Despite the tensions, a survival instinct kept her going, sometimes against the odds. Even when attacked for her views she managed to bounce back with determination. She needed to overcome timidity with temerity.

Getting the media onside with her campaign work was not easy, but she persisted and did so in what perhaps might be best described as a strategic approach. Despite her doggedness and outspokenness, she knew instinctively and experientially that it was important not to over-sensationalise. Nonetheless, there were times when she found it necessary to be somewhat sensational in order to capture attention of others to her cause.

Her charisma appeared to be an attribute that worked in her favour. She had the ability to mount convincing arguments, which was helpful in garnering funds for the work in which she believed. She demonstrated capacity to stand up for herself if warranted. For Bernadette this has sometimes meant contending with being treated badly and receiving negative responses, but she sees this as contributing to the greater good. It is important, she says, to stick to beliefs and not be compromised. Sometimes this means it is necessary to have nerves of steel.

One characteristic that Bernadette mentioned was that she does not like taking orders. It seems that she also does not like giving orders and believes that trusting people to work independently yields the best results. A principled approach enshrines her ways of working, as discussed below.

Principled Ways of Working

One of Bernadette's key principles relates to money. She did not apply for money for the sake of it. She found the competitive tendering environment particularly difficult through her own experience. She did not accept dominant paradigms such as in the Kennett era of government in Victoria—challenging the policy approaches and fighting for funding were at the heart of a principled approach. Competitive tendering had a negative effect for her when World Vision obtained a contract for the work that she had devoted much of her life to. In her view, that organisation worked *differently* and compromised and Bernadette was adamant she would not have engaged in such compromises.

She is a great believer that services should not be duplicated. Her way of developing services was based on a proposition of responding to gaps by trying to close them. She does not warm to egos that abound in the field.

Another key principle was ensuring that her organisation did not overspend on administration and she is critical of the corporate nature of organisations where spending was less circumspect. In this she never lost sight of what she was doing—and why—when others appeared to lose their moral vision.

Bernadette holds an unswerving belief that the world needs changing and recognises her own contribution to this enormous task, while acknowledging there is still work to be done. Sometimes she talks about great achievements and then recognises the mere dent in solving the problem—perhaps an inevitable paradox when working in contested and complex areas.

One issue for Bernadette is that it was not always possible to strive for the principles that she held. She learned (perhaps the hard way) that "taking on too much" was not always effective and it was better to be focused. So it seems that although acting on the belief that the world needs changing, she recognises the importance of achieving what is humanly possible. In this she took pride in the work she did, which was evidenced for her through the recognition that this gained.

Social Work as a Guiding Force: Prospects and Limitations

Bernadette is committed to radical social work and she suggests that there are lessons from her own journey for radical social workers so that they push boundaries, rather than becoming lethargic and compliant.

Ideally, she sees social workers as change agents at all levels of endeavour. They should not, she said, be mere cogs in the system. The overall formula is as follows: one starts with a problem and then works to bring about change.

Bernadette finds it regrettable that social workers do not have much clout. Social work needs to be *fired up* and less bureaucratic. It is important to speak out about injustices, particularly in a country like Australia where there is freedom to do so. She advises that social work needs to break down restrictions so social workers can speak out and lobby.

One position she takes from which social workers might take heed, particularly in a neo-liberal environment where notions of certainty and risk dominate, is to recognise that some things happen by chance and it is not always possible to predict and plan. Be in it for the long haul, she advises, and recognise that there are ups and downs. It is not realistic to expect instant gratification. It is also important to be reflective. And perhaps more than anything, social workers should not *give up*.

Empathy Across Boundaries

Although passionate about the work she did with Child Wise and angry about the harm done to others, Bernadette illustrated the capacity to walk in the shoes of others. This was demonstrated by empathy not only with victims but with perpetrators of abuse.

> I've worked with a lot of survivors of sexual abuse and sex offending, and they're very, you know, paedophiles should be put on an island and all of that, or they should never be let out of gaol, and I don't feel that. I feel compassion for sex offenders. I'm interested in the way that they think, I'm interested in the way that they operate, I'm interested in the way that they justify what they do. I don't hate them. So I don't know where that, whether that's more curiosity than compassion. I mean I certainly think there has to be protection from them, but I get really angry when the media vilify sex offenders as the biggest monsters in society because these are individuals that have issues, problems, you know, screwed-up childhoods that have led them to do something that they shouldn't be doing. They know they shouldn't be doing it, you know … so I'm one of the few moderates I think in the child protection area, or I certainly was, that had a lot of empathy, not just for the victims but for the offenders as well, but also for the family members and the impact to the family members as well.

This was also apparent in her previous work in public housing and the theme of trying to make lives better, through activist endeavours, has been consistent. She gave attention to areas where she felt she could make a difference, unlike mental health, where she perceived the system as too difficult to penetrate for change.

Bernadette also commented that she could easily work in other (but not all) fields with marginalised and vulnerable groups. This could be fostered, she suggested, by knowing her strengths, which were centred on campaigning.

Reflections on Her Lifetime of Activism: Lessons for the Field

Some of the key achievements in which Bernadette takes pride are:

- resilience to *stick it out* against the odds
- creation of a movement
- raising a son alone
- programs that she innovated.

She is not so proud, however, of *flipping the lid* too fast.

Looking back on her work, she raised the question of self-help and self-care in order to keep going. Although she worked on this, it was hard to keep going, especially as a single mother with unrelenting determination in her work. She gave heed to self-help, but balance was hard. She is adamant that she could not give up on the children but recognised the need to *recharge batteries*. She sees herself as different from other social workers, who separate out private and working lives. She now contemplates barriers to working in the present, suggesting that there is a less trusting relationship with authorities. This combines with her other concerns, including competition among non-government organisations, the entry of "corporates" into the sector and less availability of money. On quite a sad note, she reflected that having her skills no longer counts for so much.

Notwithstanding these heartfelt ponderings, Bernadette is somewhat of a pragmatist, recognising the need to be realistic about the extent of changes that come about in activist work.

Summary

A summary of core virtues for Bernadette includes resilience, determination, compassion, empathy, stubbornness, anger and lack of understanding of why others do not share her world view. Interestingly, there may be contention as to whether all of these facets would normally be seen as virtues. But if one sees virtues as fostering the capacity to achieve social change, then in a social work sense competing virtues may be important. This may challenge those who see virtues in social work as being those enshrined, but not named as such, in the Australian Association of Social Workers (AASW) Code of Ethics. This can be explained as follows.

Bernadette is largely a collegial person with good interpersonal skills and ways of working organisationally, but at the same time she is prepared to stand up for injustice in ways beyond those specified in the code. She is prepared to confront, be angry and to criticise her colleagues who work with organisational imperatives that she sees as opposing an ethical change agenda and more.

Although it is probably fair to say that most social workers wish to engage in work that is meaningful to them, she maintains a *higher* ethical stance. This is exemplified by her desire for overseas work, but a doggedness about not wanting to take any job for the sake of working overseas. Although she stated that there were other fields that she could have been as committed to, there is arguably a limit to this. Opportunities rather than plans steered her direction.

Perhaps also contradictory is her self-confessed intolerance. She could not, she told us, be tolerant when petty issues were to the forefront such as staff squabble. She quickly became certain that she did not like being a manager.

Her zealous nature appealed to some politicians and she made great gains this way. Others were not so convinced and did not lavish praise. This did not stop her from being persistent.

Two things stand out that perhaps position Bernadette differently to other social workers. One was the belief that one person can bring about change. Social workers often start as idealistic but organisational constraints diminish this. On the contrary, for Bernadette her idealism and belief in her own capacity strengthened her resolve as time went on. The second is a question of identity and most people have multiple identities. However, for Bernadette her identity became framed by Child Wise work.

From the biography it is apparent that she is an ideologue at heart and an idealist, although there were occasions when pragmatism was necessary, but only up to a point.

Conclusion

Portrayed by the media as *enemy of exploitation* and *crusader* (see the bibliography below), Bernadette's remarkable and reformational life story depicts self and social empowerment and change-oriented practice, at both local and global levels.

Along with raising her son solo, and creating a movement, Bernadette has caused significant socio-legal change in the field of child sex tourism and abuse: *There have been a lot of changes through the work that I have done and the people I've worked with have done, but not enough, not enough.*

Future social workers might well reflect on her resilience and resolve, courage and commitment, generosity and selflessness, practical, effective and innovative strategies and programs, and provocative passion.

Bibliography/References

Agora, The Magazine of la Trobe University Graduates. (2004). Crusading for children, p. 19. Agora.

Australian Centre for Leadership for Women. (2012). Bernadette McMenamin. http://www.leadershipforwomen.com.au/empowerment/leadership/bernadette-mcmenamin. Accessed 21 September 2016.

Australian Laws for Travellers: Ending child sex tourism. Information leaflet at the airport. Undated.

Child Wise. (2004). *A child wise tourism report. Traffic jam. A report on the commercial sexual exploitation of children*. Melbourne: Child Wise.

Child Wise. (2007). *Speak up about child sexual abuse: Because often they cannot. Information booklet*. Melbourne: Child Wise.

Child Wise. (undated). *Choose with care: Building child safe organisations. A national information and training program*. Melbourne: Child Wise.

ECAPT and MacKillop Family Services. (1999). *Choose with care: A recruitment guide for organisations working with children*. Melbourne: ECAPT.

Encounter (2004). *Bernadette McMenamin*. Encounter: Flinders University Magazine for Alumni and Friends, p. 20.

Frederick, John. (1999). Investigation: What Australian men do not tell their wives/Australian sex tourists: Why are they getting away with it? *Marie Claire, 45,* 50–58.

Information for Australian travellers (undated). *Do not let child abuse travel.* Information post card.

Lunn, S. (2012). Confessions of a crusader. *The Weekend Australian Magazine*, 9–10 June, pp. 13–16.

Marinos, S. (2002). Child pornography, special report. *New Idea*, 9 November, pp. 30–31.

Marinos, S. (2003). Child Abuse Report: Children for Sale. *New Idea*, 13 September, pp. 18–19.

Martyn, E. (1988). *Youth for sale: ECPAT Australia's national inquiry into the commercial sexual exploitation of children and young people in Australia.* Melbourne: ECPAT, Australia.

McMenamin, B. (2000). *National directors report. ECPAT Australia annual report 2000. Protecting children everywhere.* Melbourne: ECPAT Australia.

McMenamin, B. (2004). Letter from National Director. *Child Wise*, issue 73, Child Wise Spring Newsletter.

McMenamin, B. (2009). It takes more than money to protect our children. Opinion, *The Sunday Age 20* September, p. 17.

Minns, S. (2008). *Bernadette McMenamin* (p. 22). Vive: For women who mean business, June/July.

Outstanding graduates acknowledged (2004). *On campus: The internal newspaper of Flinders University. 13*(20), 8–21 November.

Protyniak, N. (2003). Local heroes get deserved recognition. *Herald Sun*, 18 November.

Thomas, F., & Mathews, L. (2006). *Who are the child sex tourists in Cambodia? Research study into child sex tourists in Cambodia.* Melbourne: Child Wise.

Victorian Women's Trust (2001). Bernadette McMenamin. In *Ordinary women: Extraordinary lives: Capturing the contribution of Victorian women since Federation* (p. 58). Melbourne: Victorian Women's Trust.

Vuk, J. (2000). Enemy of exploitation. War Cry, *119*(23), 3 June, p. 5. The Salvation Army.

Who (2007). Everyday beauties: Bernadette McMenamin. *Who 16* April, p. 92.

Williams, N. (2004). Thousands of paedophiles travel for sex. *Advertiser*, 28 October.

Chapter 9
You Roll up Your Sleeves and You Help, and Work with People—Robyn Miller

Manohar Pawar and Sharlene Nipperess

Dr. Robyn Miller is a social worker and family therapist with over 30 years experience in the field. She began her career as a social work practitioner at Catholic Family Welfare in 1980 and attained the demanding leadership positions of Principal Practitioner in 2006, and Director and Chief Practitioner of the Department of Human Services (DHS) in Victoria in 2014. Robyn has been a member of the Victorian Child Death Review Committee for the past nine years. She has worked in the community sector, local government and child protection and at the Bouverie Centre, Victoria's Family Institute at La Trobe University, as a senior clinician and consultant. She has published several articles and chapters and authored the *Best Interests Series* for the DHS. Robyn is noted for her innovative practice with children and families where there is complex and trans-generational trauma. She supports and inspires professionals to always keep the best interests of children at the centre of decisions. By providing valuable practice leadership to social workers within and beyond the department, Robyn has effected positive change in the lives of many Victorians. She was the recipient of the inaugural Robin Clark memorial Ph.D. scholarship in 2004 and a Robin Clark Memorial Award in 2010 for her inspirational leadership in the field.

M. Pawar (✉)
Charles Sturt University, Wagga Wagga, Australia
e-mail: mpawar@csu.edu.au

S. Nipperess
RMIT University, Melbourne, Australia
e-mail: sharlene.nipperess@rmit.edu.au

M. Pawar et al. (eds.), *Empowering Social Workers*,
DOI 10.1007/978-981-10-3809-9_9

The Early Years

Robyn Miller was born in Melbourne in 1958 to Joan and Ray Clements. She was the second child in a family of six children, which included her elder brother Peter and her younger siblings Danny, Cathy, Sean and Joanne. Robyn describes a very close and loving family.

The influence of Robyn's mother, maternal grandmother and great-grandmother is strong. Her great-grandmother was from a well-to-do family but she married a bullock driver called Donaldson. He was a bit of a larrikin according to Robyn, and she remembers lots of stories of him and other family characters as she was growing up. Robyn's great-grandmother was rejected by her wealthy family for marrying Donaldson but she proved to be *a resourceful, strong woman* who managed to raise nine children on her own after her husband died.

Blanche, Robyn's grandmother, was one of these nine children. Robyn has very fond memories of Blanche: *She lived till she was 90, but was just this wonderful, gorgeous, loving, warm, funny woman who I adored.* Blanche married Frank Upton and they had six children. Joan was their fourth child and Robyn's mother. They grew up in North Fitzroy in Melbourne and it was a wonderful family with *a lot of joy, a lot of characters, a lot of music, a lot of dancing* but not a lot of money. Robyn recalls that they had a *terrific love for children and valuing of family*. Frank and Blanche met after Frank came back from the First World War. He had been at Gallipoli in Turkey and Fromelles in France. He had a stable job during the Depression and worked for the Royal Children's Hospital for over forty years.

Robyn was part of a large, extended, but very well connected family. She had 30 first cousins and notes that they *would always have Christmas together ... all of the key celebrations, and food was very important, having a singalong, having a dance, and a very Irish, very Irish tradition.*

Robyn notes that there was a lot of fun in her mother's household while she was growing up, but this contrasted somewhat with her father's family. Her father Ray and his brother Frank also grew up in inner Melbourne in the suburb of Collingwood. Their mother and father both worked in the boot factories, but their father *was a bit of a scoundrel and not a nice man at all*, according to Robyn, and as a result Ray *grew up with a fair bit of shame and trauma*. She feels her father was attracted to her mother's close-knit family, which was always open and welcoming—on Sunday evenings it was always open house. All the relatives would visit for cold meat and salad, stories and dancing. Robyn has strong memories of growing up in a *stable, safe environment* that came predominantly from her mother's family.

Joan and Ray met at St. John's in Clifton Hill, a Catholic youth organisation. Robyn notes that her grandmother, Blanche, was not Catholic, but Frank was. Nevertheless, Blanche sent Robyn's mother and her siblings *looking beautiful* to Mass every Sunday. While Blanche did not go to Mass and nor did Frank, they always went at Christmas and all of the children went to Catholic schools. Robyn identifies that *nobody ever had a very ... fundamental view of Catholicism; it was always very inclusive, there was a respect.*

Joan and Ray got married and within a year they had their first child, Peter, and then Robyn was born 13 months later. They bought a house in West Preston/East Coburg. At that time Joan's mother Blanche was running a milk bar in Northcote and so she provided a lot of support to Robyn's mum, who was 20 when she had her first child. Robyn's dad *worked around the clock.* He did an apprenticeship in the boot trade but then went to work for Bulla Cream and at times had two or three jobs. He worked for Four'n Twenty pies—*an archetypal working class upbringing*—but eventually he started his own business. Robyn recalls him being a really hard worker and this work ethic was instilled early in all of the children, as was the *notion of how lucky we were.* On the other hand, his trauma and use of alcohol concerned and pained all family members.

Joan was at home full time with the children, so it was a very traditional arrangement according to Robyn, and at times *a tough gig* for her mother. Robyn notes that:

> My mum was a great mother, just fantastic, and she's 78 now, still very connected and has been a rock and just very, very sensible, very loving, very warm, and progressive thinking … My mum had it down pat, and so did my grandmother: high warmth, low hostility and clear boundaries.

Joan made sure that even though there was not very much money, all the kids had opportunities.

Robyn remembers a childhood that was full of freedom and fun. Their house was on the Merri Creek so, even though they lived in suburban Melbourne, beyond their back fence were a couple of paddocks where horses were kept, and the creek. Robyn says her mother:

> was very relaxed, so she wouldn't worry that we were walking along the fence or climbing over fences; she wasn't a "nervous Nellie". So we were able to take risks as kids, we were always swinging on the willow trees down there, we'd come back full of mud and dirt.

They spent a lot of time with their cousins building cubby houses and engaging in imaginary play. In addition to the freedom of outside play, Robyn recalls other opportunities she had when growing up, such as learning the piano and Irish dancing, for which she became Victorian champion.

As eldest girl, it was expected that Robyn would help out with the younger children. There was a strong ethic in the family that all of the children were required to help, but *there was something about being eldest girl.* From the earliest days Robyn can remember that it was her role to bath all of the kids on Saturday night, but she notes that *I wasn't overburdened because my grandmother would come nearly every week and help Mum clean and cook.*

The birth of Joanne, the youngest of Ray and Joan's children, was particularly significant and Robyn describes it as *a defining moment in my life.* Joanne was born with Down Syndrome and Robyn recalls her paternal grandmother saying, "Oh God, I wish God would take her. I wish God would take her". Robyn remembers a fierce reaction from deep within her: *What do you mean, God take her*? Robyn remembers, *I just was furious that she'd even have thought that she'd want this little baby to die, just because she'd got Down Syndrome*. It was a confusing experience for Robyn and her siblings, because on the one hand they were joyous that they had a baby sister but on the other Robyn recalls her father crying. This life event initiated her values of right to life.

School Education and Becoming a Social Worker

Robyn's father left school at 14, and despite being *a really smart man*, his family could not afford for him to stay in school past year eight. Joan also left school at year eight, although at that time it was not uncommon for girls to leave early. But education for Robyn and her siblings was never questioned.

Robyn went to the local Catholic primary school, St. Raphael's in West Preston, and then to Santa Maria College in Northcote, an all-girls Catholic school run by Good Samaritan nuns. According to Robyn she had very nurturing teachers: *I loved school, I always enjoyed it, and I made really good friends, laughed a lot, had a lot of fun*. It was at secondary school that one of the nuns, Sister Placid, identified that Robyn had advanced empathy and suggested psychology as a potential career path.

Robyn held a variety of leadership positions at school and she recalls that in year 12 when she was school captain she was in charge of uniform inspection, which she *hated doing, but it was again, how do you work this out to be a win-win*? She organised a number of students to be at the main train and tram stops to forewarn students of the uniform inspection, and to provide spare blazers and hats if necessary, *so by the time they got to school no one would fail the inspection*.

Somewhere around the end of year 12 Robyn began to think of youth work as a possible career. She applied for a position at the Social Welfare Institute, for which she was successful, but then someone, perhaps a teacher, asked whether she had heard of social work. They explained that social work was much broader than youth work and that there were opportunities for working in a range of fields. Robyn thought that sounded good, so she started looking for information on social work courses. Eventually she found the PIT (Preston Institute of Technology) course, which at that stage was very new.[1] Robyn liked the fact that it was a four-year degree and she commenced studies in 1976.

She says it was a very good, balanced course and she had the opportunity to study a range of subjects, including philosophy, biology, social biology and legal studies, as well as psychology for four years. According to Robyn *the foundational framework was a systems approach* and she remembers being taught a year of family therapy in third year. She did a placement every year and Robyn describes

[1]PIT was the second social work course in Melbourne (the first being at Melbourne University). PIT was merged with the Royal Melbourne Institute of Technology (RMIT) in 1992.

these as key learning experiences. In her final year she was placed at Span Community House at the Brotherhood of St. Laurence, being involved in social action with older people.

At the same time Robyn was involved in a great deal of volunteer work. In her first year, and throughout her degree, she volunteered on a St. Vincent de Paul soup van. She says: *I knew that territory from all my family stories, and the pubs that they would talk about, The Champion and The Rob Roy on the two corners of Gertrude Street and Brunswick Street Fitzroy ... I loved the characters, and again great teachers.*

Robyn believes that she learned and became committed to a relationship-based approach working on the van. She also volunteered for about three years, one night a week, with Connie Benn on the children's program, a project of the Brotherhood of St. Laurence. She was engaged in a number of activities with the children, including attending camps. It was an empowerment model and Robyn notes *for me as a young social work student it just fitted with those social justice values that I was already imbued with perfectly.*

During holidays, when Robyn was 19 and 20 years old, she participated in a volunteer program hosted by the Melbourne Catholic Church and Australian Volunteers Abroad, which involved flying twice to Kanabea, New Guinea, to assist remote communities to access education and health services. Robyn recognises her *love of travel, adventure and learning about different cultures stems from that life changing opportunity*. Finally, she volunteered teaching English to Vietnamese refugees at the Maribyrnong Reception Centre, as it was known then. She notes that *again, the gift in that was the teaching they gave us about the experience of asylum seekers, and my horror of what is happening in this country today around the misinformation and lies.*

Her volunteer experiences *were as important to me in my social work training as any other theoretical paradigms I was given.* She also recognises the role of her paid work as a waitress, which she did through university to pay the rent, for by this stage she had moved out of home.

Robyn met her husband—Robert Miller—while volunteering in New Guinea and together they have had five children: Patrick, Chris, Sean, Bridie and Joseph. She notes: *He's very important in my life and has always been incredibly supportive of my professional work.* Robert is a teacher and Robyn notes that they share the same values and Irish Catholic background.

Social Work Practice and Further Study

Robyn completed her social work degree in 1979 and commenced practice in 1980 as a pregnancy counsellor at Catholic Family Welfare Bureau. She recalls that financial support for *unmarried mothers*, as they were referred to then, had not been available that long and there was huge pressure for women to adopt their babies. She notes that *although it was a Catholic institution there was strong support for women choosing to keep their babies. So my role was to support the women*. She was about 22 years old and she remembers *the grief, loss, trauma, often rape ... sexual abuse* that these women experienced, the pressure to move to St. Joseph's on Grattan Street opposite the Royal Women's Hospital, a home run for unmarried mothers by the Josephite nuns and again *the fierce determination that no one would force these girls to do anything they didn't want to do*. Robyn notes that it was very complex work and she learned a lot from the other therapists in the organisation, but *I do remember going home and crying my eyes out several nights to Rob, just with the sadness of it*.

Their first son, Patrick, was born in 1982 and Robyn returned to work in mid-1983, to a new role at Melbourne City Council and Catholic Care. She was a family counsellor and co-director of a children's centre in North Carlton, in charge of a unit that was for children whose families required respite care. Robyn recalls it *meant that young parents in the high-rise flats in the local area could get a break when they needed it and not wait until ... things had deteriorated*. Essentially it was a counselling role with the families of the children who were using the respite service, but she managed the childcare workers and the carers, set up systems and introduced more reflective practice and group supervision. Again the work was quite complex, with children disclosing abuse while they were in the respite care or in the kinder program. Robyn notes: *that period was pretty challenging. I learnt a lot. I learnt a lot about managing staff, about managing a service and working as a team*. It was flexible and worked well with family life—she had her second son, Chris, in 1984—and she returned to the role after his birth. However, it also proved unsafe at times. Robyn remembers being forced to leave her own home due to violent threats from male clients. She has reflected on these incidents and notes:

> what I learnt was fear and … I kept thinking, God I'm lucky. I've got all these organisational people helping me … I've got strong family to go home to. I've got a good husband. I've got all these positives. What must it be like to be a woman that sits there who's a victim of violence that is terrified night after night?

Robyn commenced her third role at the Fitzroy Council as a family counsellor after she had her third son, Sean, in 1987. It was in the Social Planning Office—she says *I hadn't gone very far from the Carlton flats to the Fitzroy flats*. It fitted well with the multidisciplinary approach that made sense to Robyn, and had a human rights approach to developing social services. Like all her roles, Robyn *loved it*. She worked closely with the Maternal and Child Health nursing team and attended the playgroups because:

> a lot of these women were scared stiff to see a counsellor, but all had some complex problems around violence. So what we learnt to do, I'd go to the play groups and hang out and they could see I didn't have two heads and I was down to earth and approachable so I would do a lot of work, engagement, through there … so my role was a lot of outreach.

At this time she also started doing a lot of work in child protection. Mandatory reporting was just being introduced and the Social Planning Office had a strong view that the community was responsible for child protection and the risk with mandatory reporting would be that all responsibility would be deferred to the DHS.

Robyn notes that for the first ten years of her career she had *never been on the mandated side of the fence.*

In 1990 Robyn commenced a two-year family therapy course at the Bouverie Centre, while pregnant with her fourth child. Bridie was born in December of the first year and went with Robyn every week during the second year of the course. Robyn says it *was the best move I ever made.* Although all previous jobs were so rich in terms of learning, for Robyn the move to Bouverie was important, as it helped to integrate her practice with theoretical developments and to enhance her confidence.

At the same time, even though Robyn had a young baby, she still needed to work, so she took on some after-hours child protection work. Again it fitted in with her family life and she remembers *it was the best experience.* It was the first time she had been the mandated worker. Although she loved it, she knew she could not do it forever. It was short-term crisis intervention:

> so it was enormously rich learning because I'd go from the most incredible—you know, things where people have been murdered or children have been harmed … and then going to Bouverie the next day and explaining to people who were working in nice, safe, middle class mental health jobs.

In 1992 Robyn was offered a position at the Bouverie Centre after she graduated with a Graduate Diploma in Family Therapy, and she took it despite being sad to leave her community role in Fitzroy. She had developed significant experience in sexual assault/family violence work. At Bouverie there were a number of small teams and Robyn became a member of the sexual abuse team. Although she notes it *was a terrible name* it was about *critiquing the traditional therapeutic ways of working with families where there'd been sexual abuse.* At Bouverie she started teaching in the family therapy course and did a lot of supervision. But what stood out, as a real growth area for her, was that she started doing a lot more clinical work with offenders. The specialist family therapy work at Bouverie was informed by feminist theory and was largely long term in nature. Robyn identifies that it was a *rich experience in terms of learning* and she began publishing some of this work with her colleagues.

At the same time she commenced work in private practice. At Bouverie the staff were involved in direct clinical work, supervision, consultation and training, so this is what she did in her private practice as well. There were about a dozen organisations that she worked with regularly, including maternal and child health, Methodist Ladies College school counselling team and the Alfred Hospital social work department. Again, this work was part time and fitted well with her family life. In 1995 Robyn gave birth to her fifth child, Joseph.

In 1997 she completed a Master of Family Therapy and in 2004 decided to leave Bouverie, after 12 years. The DHS had developed a program called Take Two, which was the state-wide mental health service for children in child protection or out-of-home care. Robyn was approached to be involved, which precipitated her decision to leave Bouverie. At the same time it was suggested that she ought to be doing a Ph.D. and, given that the Take Two program offered a scholarship, she applied and was awarded the inaugural Robyn Clarke memorial Ph.D. scholarship. She commenced her studies in 2004 and was recently awarded her Ph.D.

In 2005 Robyn experienced a health crisis that had a significant impact on her and her family. It was found that she had a tumour on her ovary, which was subsequently removed. At that time *a shadow on her kidney* was noticed and six weeks later she was back in hospital to have the cancer removed from her kidney. This was a huge shock, as Robyn felt that she had *always been so fit and well and healthy*, but while she was in hospital recovering, Gill Callister from the DHS rang her and offered her a job as Principal Practitioner. Gill wanted to build a culture of reflective practice and Robyn remembers *lying there thinking and all of a sudden the sun shone and it was like "Yes, I think this is right"*.

From 2006 to 2012 Robyn worked as Principal Practitioner within the Children, Youth and Families Division of the DHS. In December 2012 she became Chief Practitioner Human Services. Initially she was not involved in managing other people—it was a stand-alone role, working with everyone in the department. Her role was to inspire good practice, to build the culture of reflective practice, improve the quality of decision making inside child protection and develop research. Robyn notes *the job description was very big*. Over time, with additional support and funding from the department, Robyn grew a team of people and the *operating model in child protection changed* from having less experienced people carrying the cases to the more experienced people taking responsibility for complex cases. The tradition had been the more experienced a worker got, the further they moved away from practice. The new approach has dramatically improved the retention rate inside child protection according to Robyn. *So, you know, rolling up my sleeves really is how I framed it and saying, "Well, yeah, I'll do that one" and thinking "Well, what's the use having a principal practitioner if you're not prepared to work on the most challenging cases?"*

During this time Robyn developed the Best Interests Case Practice Model and has co-authored a range of specialist resources that have been taken up in Australia and overseas. Her Ph.D. thesis, "'Walking the same talk': Promoting cultural reform in the Victorian Child Protection and Family Services through the Best Interests Case Practice Model", explores in detail the reform work that she has led within the department. When reflecting on her work, Robyn is proud that she has continued to work *from those very first principles of respect, you do no harm, you treat people well* and she notes:

> we talk a lot about vicarious trauma; I don't think we talk enough about the vicarious joy. When you've … been privileged to be present in the depths of their despair and you see this incredible human spirit of courage, of strength, of, you know, sheer guts often to keep going in the worst of circumstances. It's extraordinary, you know.

In recognition of Robyn's practice leadership, the Robin Clark Memorial Award was conferred on her in 2010 for her inspirational leadership in the field.

Analysis of Qualities/Character

Some of the qualities and character building that stand out in Robyn Miller's practice-focused biography are discussed below. Her statement *I think of who I am now as who I was then*, seems to suggest that she already had certain qualities that were/are conducive to professional social work practice that she has been engaged in for over three decades. It is interesting to explore what those qualities are, though they are not presented in any particular order.

Valuing Family

To Robyn, family (broadly defined: any association of members who live like family) is the centre of the universe. Having been brought up in a large and extended family, with a lot of cousins, aunts and uncles and grandmothers who frequently gathered, celebrated events and often supported each other in times of need, Robyn strongly valued family as a tradition and a crucial source of security, love, joy and fun, singing and dancing in the spirit of Irish tradition, and the foundation for further development. As Robyn notes, *the valuing of joy and celebration in my family that, despite the difficulties, was always there and [we] had enormous freedom as kids.*

As a growing child, Robyn remembers receiving enough warmth, love and security from her parents; gaining insights by listening to stories of relatives; and having necessary opportunities for development, though without a lot of money. Valuing the centrality of family and its roles and functions is reflected in Robyn's practice life, which has mostly revolved around understanding and contributing to creating families in which all their members have what they are normally expected to have. Robyn's faith or belief in the family as a nurturing unit is very strong: *I was genuinely interested in the stories and in people's lives and in understanding the family history'*. As she notes:

> I suppose when I think about children in out-of-home care now I think about the quality of their experience and love, what are they receiving in terms of they've got every right to have all the good things in life. And that doesn't mean just food and shelter, it means opportunities to do the sort of things that we all want for our kids and that we all had growing up.

Respect, Courtesy and Relationship

As Robyn was raised in a large and extended family, basic human qualities such as being respectful, courteous and polite to each other were developed in her from the very beginning. Knowing and relating to all the extended family members was part of learning to develop relationships. Robyn notes: *because our family culture was very much you are polite and you're very respectful, and always being respectful to the relations, and there were a lot of them ... But always, very clearly you were never rude and you were always welcoming of everybody.*

From the earliest days Robyn learnt that the *best way to often connect with people was just to be courteous and welcoming.* When she practised these in one of the workplaces, it *broke all the rules because in a formal psychiatric mental health facility that wasn't sort of the normal thing at the time.* She remembers some people laughing when she offered to get the client a cup of tea. Here the "relationship" does not refer to the "professional relationship" in social work practice, but the way we relate and connect to people in our day-to-day affairs. It is the basic humanness to connect or touch with people we interact with. To Robyn such a basic relationship—respect and courtesy—is important in professional practice.

Religion: Social Justice, Equality, Rights and Inclusiveness

Robyn studied in a Catholic school and her parents regularly took their children to attend weekly Mass. She was influenced by a not strictly Catholic ethos, but Christian ethos, such as *look after the underdog and you have got a duty of care.* Words often rang in her head, like: *if you are blessed in life, to whom much is given much is expected.* Robyn was in the choir—had a *strong parish sort of church connection, but strong sense of community, knew neighbours and people around and always valued them.* Through this process, Robyn internalised the values of valuing everybody, regardless of their station in life; all are equal; and the notion of not getting ahead of yourself. Robyn remembers school retreats and how she was inspired:

> I remember hanging up quotes in my bedroom … while someone is not fed, while someone is in prison … none of us are free, you know, that sense of that interconnectedness. And the duty of care, I suppose, as a humane society … so I suppose I was very drawn to that and so I was no goody-two-shoes at school.

Robyn was also taught about Buddhism and Hinduism, and respect for other religions. It was not just preaching. She heard stories of how her grandmother cared for a brother who was homeless. Her grandmother fed, washed and gave him freshly cleaned clothes and did not look down upon him because he was homeless. Robyn said, *I think that strong sense of social justice was just grown into me from my grandmother.* She remembers that her father *supported the unions and was a lifetime Labor voter, and he would stick up for the underdog.* In his workplace, when a worker bullied a homosexual worker, Robyn's father intervened to stop the bullying. Her family was open about such matters.

When her sister was born with Down syndrome, Robyn's paternal grandmother was not able to accept the reality, and the doctor advised Robyn's mother to relinquish the baby to an institution. Robyn was furious about such reactions and said, *I think my fierce determination that you respect the rights of everybody, something galvanised in me at that point and I've no doubt that that was a turning point in me. She's got every right to have a good life.* Robyn's mother, with her own good sense, simply rejected such advice and proudly raised the baby with dignity. As a student in year nine, Robyn wrote on the rights of children with disability and presented it to her class.

She cannot tolerate any racist comments and she feels fierce about Aboriginal history and the current context:

> The appreciation of culture particularly for Aboriginal children and families has been a passion of mine in the role. The over representation of Aboriginal children in out-of-home care is of great concern to me and has driven my efforts to contribute to different practice reforms. Particularly in a statutory context, the importance of a rights-based approach and of practitioners having deep respect and knowledge about the experience of colonisation and of the Stolen Generation is crucial.

Robyn has mingled with people from multicultural backgrounds. She said, *so that valuing of people regardless of their station in life, I suppose, was embedded in family and at school really. So I got a strong dose of that.*

Volunteering

Robyn undertook a lot of voluntary work while at school and university, for a number of years, which shows her interest in helping others. She undertook voluntary work in Papua New Guinea (PNG) and offered services in the areas of education and health. She taught English to Vietnamese refugees, helped organise a soup van and later led it as a president, and worked for the children's program of the Brotherhood of St Laurence that followed an empowerment approach. Robyn also raised funds, particularly for Kanabea, after returning from PNG.

To Robyn volunteering was a means to an end—developing meaningful relationships with people. In fact, her relationship-based practice approach originated from her years of voluntary work.

Tune into People—Leadership

During her school years Robyn demonstrated her leadership qualities and ability to relate to her peers. She was class captain often and she also was on the school representative council. Many girls used to confide in her and she organised help for them. She said, *I loved being with people and liked working with other girls at school.* Robyn remembers organising the Good Friday appeal with other girls and raised $3000 by knocking on doors. She set up lunchtime clubs, homework, chess clubs and so on, and tried to include people who were being left out. She was exposed to shared and collaborative leadership styles. One of the teachers told Robyn that she had advanced empathy and that meant she could tune into people. She received an award (Santa Maria Old Collegians) for the girl with the most influence. As stated earlier, she was also president of the soup van.

As a social work practitioner, Robyn has tuned into several client groups and colleagues in a number of organisations and she has effectively worked with children, women and men. These qualities have made her a leader in practice, research, teaching and training. Her gravitation to practice has taken Robyn to the highest leadership position: Chief Practitioner and Director of the Office of Professional Practice in the DHS.

Adventure, Courage and Fear

Robyn says she wanted adventure in life and has loved adventurous activities:

> I loved adventure, always have loved adventure, and always loved going on all the fast rides … because I loved going fast, and I loved going on a boat … I didn't have a lot of fear in me. I always loved, I didn't feel ever scared going around the back streets … and then people said, "Aren't you scared of going?" I said, "No, it's so interesting." I remember going into the boarding houses and you know, when I look back I think God I don't know that I'd want my daughter doing that at that age; but I didn't ever feel frightened because of the relationships we formed with people on the street and the teams that worked together.

Robyn travelled in a small plane to undertake volunteer activities in the Gulf Province in PNG, to provide education and health services in isolated areas. She helped to deliver babies and learned to give injections.

As a practitioner, Robyn has worked with clients who were living with abusive and violent partners and sometimes her decisions and interventions led to life-threatening situations. This caused anxiety and fear to the extent that her family had to move out of their home and security arrangements were made at their workplaces. Robyn said:

> I don't know whether I needed any more empathy for women who are exposed to violence … you think you know what fear is but I didn't have a clue what fear was until I'd experienced that. And the importance of worker safety issues, the importance of understanding offenders. So I became much more interested, I suppose, in thinking about how offenders tick and that we needed more of that knowledge in training.

Robyn's current work often involves deciphering complicated cases, taking decisions and presenting in court; all have a sense of adventure and require courage to lead.

Learning: Reflective Practice, Research and Enhanced Confidence

Robyn's biography and practice career show how she was eager to learn and how she has kept continuously learning through her reflections on practice, formal training and university courses, research and writing on practice, and by both offering and receiving supervision. In the social work course, she says, she had so much to learn. As a practitioner: *I learnt an enormous amount from the other therapists at the organisation at the time, so it was a rich organisation to be in, really, for professional development and counselling skills, because there was a strong bent there.*

According to Robyn, practitioners do not need to know everything if they are willing to learn from their clients. She said:

> I always say now, your clients, your families are your greatest teachers; they'll teach you … don't feel like you've got to know everything. None of us know everything. Sometimes I think none of us know anything in some situations. You have to negotiate a way, find a way through.

In addition to her practice with clients, as a co-director of the family support program Robyn was conscious about how she *learnt about managing staff, about managing a service and working as a team.*

When Robyn began family therapy training at the Bouverie Centre, she felt it was the best move she ever made. She reflected on her learning:

> I say that but all of these jobs were so rich in terms of learning. I don't regret anything I've done. It's just been such a good experience and such a rich learning in everything I've done. But Bouverie was able to consolidate and give me some theoretical underpinnings and refine my therapeutic practice and give me more confidence about my own views on what I knew was a good way to treat people and I knew was a good way to engage. But they gave me more professional and theoretical language to describe what I was doing and I learnt new things too.
>
> I'm sure by the end of that two years I'd increased my confidence around what I knew to be good practice. It gave me a language and a depth and a knowledge base and some evidence base … and if you read the best interest case practice model it's all that same stuff. You know, ecological, systemic, developmentally informed, strength-based approach. Still forensically astute … all of those things. Gender, applying the feminist critique.

While at the Bouverie, through private practice Robyn provided consultancy and supervision to dozens of organisations, which she found interesting because she *felt like a bee taking pollen here and there and she learnt from everywhere she went.* Later she completed her doctoral research on her practice relating to the Best Interests Case Practice Model, which is based on the integration of knowledge from research and critical reflection (Miller 2014).

As a chief Practitioner of Human Services and director of professional practice, Robyn said: *such a rich environment and, you know, all sorts of experiences I've been able to learn from ... through that engagement ... around the state but also with other states and nationally and internationally.*

Robyn emphasised the importance of continuous learning: *people think they can do a degree and then think they're right to practice. You know, you've got to keep learning and keep up.*

Being Innovative and Change Oriented

Closely connected to learning, reflective practice and research is being innovative, which is important in social work practice (Pawar 2014). Robyn has demonstrated well the quality of being innovative in her practice. Innovation may also often require close and critical observation. Robyn said: *I've always been astute around observational stuff; it just comes with me; (laughs), I was just born with that.* When she goes on home visits, she always looks for something positive to comment on. Although the offending parent may be a problem in the child protection context, it is important to look at the *good along with the bad and ugly* of such a parent in the overall family context so as to empower the individual and family rather than just pathologising.

To Robyn, the Bouverie Centre looked like a middle-class mental health clinic, which did not have a culture of home visits and that was an important initiative. Similarly, the Indigenous family therapy network and specialised training was innovative and an important initiative. Robyn's efforts to link the *head quarters to ground quarters* were reformative and innovative in the given context. Changing the linearity of risk assessment to circularity of relationship-based practice, engagement, learning and relearning to change for the better was Robyn's innovation and change (Miller 2012). Activating the legal process to appeal against court cases was also an important innovation.

Diligence

Robyn internalised the ethos of hard work early from her parents. Her father had to work many shifts and for several hours at odd times, holding on to a series of jobs to meet the needs of the large family, and that was a tough gig for her mother, who devoted her life to raising five children and doing all the domestic chores.

Throughout her career, Robyn has always worked hard. Raising five children, doing part-time work, sometimes at odd hours in night shifts, flexibly adapting to the changing family circumstances, undertaking intensive study and private practice needs more than hard-working ability. Robyn said:

> I have always worked hard, but the nature and intensity of work in the current practice leadership job …

> I still sweat when I go to court and I prepare like anything … many times stayed up half the night because you've got to know your stuff and you've got to be well prepared and the files are thick and you've got to be up to cross-examination … but it's not frustrating because you've got to be accountable and it's a rigorous system and so it should be.

> I nearly left … and I said "I just can't, it's just something not right". I've never worked so hard in my life as for the last eight years; I feel like we've sprinted, because it was such a fertile time for change and working with all the agencies was so important.

Drawing on the wisdom of years of hard work, Robyn said, *You roll up your sleeves and you help people; you work with them and earn your stripes.*

Passion and Commitment

Robyn's hard work speaks for her passion and commitment. Her life story and career trajectory clearly bring out her passion for and commitment to practice with children and families through her best interests case practice model. She was really passionate about getting this model up in DHS and getting the principal practitioners' team up in various parts of Victoria. Despite many of her achievements, she always feels there is so much to do. Passion for Robyn is about always making things practical. She often wonders about how to make the practice more family centred and friendly, organising case conferences at home or at the child's residential unit. Robyn is passionate about debunking some of the myths in practice such as *you cannot engage an involuntary client*. Wherever Robyn worked she found it hard to leave, as she had enjoyed work so much. She is passionate about and committed to people, and relationships with people. She is keen to take practice to where people are, rather than office-based settings: *there was always in me a strong determination to stay connected to the ground ... to practice on the ground and I've kept that up.*

Humility

Robyn appeared humble by nature. Despite such enviable qualities and achievements, when she was asked to consider the principal practitioner assignment, her response was that the office should approach some more famous people, as she had not published much. When asked what is she proud of, Robyn's response was a long pause and then she said: *I think that I've held a genuine position with people and that seeing myself as being of service, you know that regardless of where I've worked... I think I've stayed humble, in a nutshell.*

After another pause, her further response was as:

> Well, you know, holding on to the humility of what you don't know, that you're not practising from ego … because I think to practise well … you do have to ride both ponies … the humility to be open to what you don't know and views or judgements you might be making that actually aren't quite fair because of A, B, C and D. But equally, the sort of courage and wherewithal to stand your ground and do what you need to do when you do know something's not right.

When this job was offered, Robyn was on the hospital bed and she recalls what she thought at that time and those thoughts show what she does and does not know: *So, I've never had a five-year plan, I've never had an ambition to do ... anything in particular. It's been like very organic and it just felt right ... because I thought "I'm lousy on computers, I'm lousy on budgets but I know about practice".*

Appreciating and Caring for Colleagues/Employees and Team Building

Under Robyn's able practice leadership, humane approaches have been developed to support a range of practitioners at various levels, and their work is appreciated. This is showing heartening results. But Robyn says, *None of this is me and a whole lot of people are working on these issues*, showing how she recognises all staff members' contributions. About workers, Robyn says the following:

> I think that whole thing around recognising people's professionalism as social workers, they come into the field because they love kids, want to do the right thing by families. We're not police. How do you harness that? There's so much goodwill inside the profession and inside the department and reclaiming … that practice ethos and challenging some of the, what we call the "bureaucratisation" of social work.

Robyn recognises that there are good social workers everywhere and it is important to write about their good practice in terms of creative and beautiful things they do. She said, *You've got to hold on to and nurture your workforce*. Although hers was a sole position, she took the initiative and joined teams and formed teams, and said, *there's good people everywhere; you've just got to connect with them*. Thus she joined forces with good people within the department. She praised her colleagues as extraordinary leaders.

Robyn suggests having a self-care plan for workers, as they work with a lot of very painful, traumatic, dark issues and it needs to be balanced with positive things in life—exercise, meditation or whatever connects to positives.

Wicked Humour

Robyn said that she has a wicked sense of humour, which she got from her family and it is helpful in her work:

> I think that's been a big part of me coping with my work really … that ability to see the ridiculous in the most bizarre and serious circumstances. I can often see the theatre in it and the sense of the ridiculous. And that stood me in good stead many times, because I often think, "Oh, people wouldn't believe what I'm doing right now, or what I'm hearing, or what I'm …

Humour is used as a mechanism for self-care, but the importance of fun and laughter generally was stated often by Robyn. Her stories were frequently recounted with laughter but the humour was often pointed towards herself and the ridiculous, rather than being directed towards clients or colleagues.

Gender

Robyn referred to her family as a traditional family, as her mother was home raising five children with a lot of love, caring and warmth. She said her teachers, who were nuns, and also her social work teachers, were very strong feminists and she was aware of the feminist critique and did not want to marry early. She said her husband was very supportive to her in raising their children and in facilitating her career trajectory:

> He has always been incredibly supportive of my professional work: I was very lucky, I had a fantastic partner who cooked, who would clean nappies, who bathed babies. And I remember my mother coming and saying "Oh you're so lucky he's bathing the baby". And I'm saying, "Well of course he does; why shouldn't he?"

Her husband is a school teacher and able to take school holidays and this made a huge difference to the quality of their family life. Nowhere did Robyn present gender as an issue, or struggles related to feminism, though while working with offending parents she used a clear feminist-informed model.

Love

Love was a concept that Robyn used frequently. Rather than the expression of an individualised, intimate love, the terms *love* and *loving* were used to describe her feelings about certain experiences. For example, she said a number of times that she *loved school* and her varied work roles. Being loving was something that she also valued highly. She described her grandmother as *loving*, her mother as *very loving* and noted that her family had a *terrific love for children*. She also expressed her love in relation to the people with whom she worked.

Conclusion

The interview with Robyn Miller demonstrates a number of qualities that were largely developed in her family of origin and have proven to be very significant in her social work career. Characteristics such as humility—strongly connected to her belief in her good luck—her strong work ethic, her compassion and empathy for people less fortunate than herself, and her fierce determination to advocate for the rights of children and families were developed early and are evident throughout her practice. Other attributes such as her commitment to relationship-based practice, innovative and change-oriented practice, team work and valuing colleagues and feminist practice, were developed later in her social work studies and in her practice in a range of organisations.

References

Miller, R. (2012). *Best interests case practice model: Specialist practice resource*. Melbourne: Victorian Government Department of Human Services.

Miller, R. (2014). *'Walking the same talk': Promoting cultural reform in Victorian child protection and family services through the best interests case practice model* (Ph.D. thesis). Melbourne: La Trobe University.

Pawar, M. (2014). *Social challenges and policy innovations by social workers in Australia* (CSD Working Paper 14–10). St. Louis, MO: Washington University, Center for Social Development. http://csd.wustl.edu/Publications/Documents/WP14-10.pdf

Chapter 10
Hunger for Movement and Action—Sue Vardon, AO

Manohar Pawar and Sue King

Sue Vardon spent 23 years as a chief executive (CE) in federal and state government agencies. She has an honorary doctorate from the University of South Australia and has been an adjunct professor at both Canberra University and the University of South Australia and was the inaugural Telstra Australian Business Woman of the Year in 1995. She was educated as a social worker at the University of New South Wales and worked in local government in NSW, both metropolitan and country. She held senior positions in the NSW Department for Community Services before moving to South Australia to become the Director General of Community Welfare. This was followed by the CE of the Office of Public Sector Reform, the Public Service Commissioner and the CE of the Department for Correctional Services in South Australia. She was the inaugural CE of Centrelink, which was established in 1997, and her last position was CE of the South Australian Department for Families and Communities, bringing together housing, disability, domiciliary care and family services. Included in this work was her role as State Recovery Co-ordinator and Chair of the National Community Services and Disability Administrators Disaster Recovery Group. Sue's inspirational story demonstrates her strength of character and shrewdness in choice of strategy.

M. Pawar (✉)
School of Humanities and Social Sciences, Charles Sturt University,
Wagga Wagga, Australia
e-mail: mpawar@csu.edu.au

S. King
University of South Australia, Adelaide, Australia
e-mail: sue.king@unisa.edu.au

M. Pawar et al. (eds.), *Empowering Social Workers*,
DOI 10.1007/978-981-10-3809-9_10

Early Life

Suzanne Sharon Vardon was born in 1948 and is popularly known as Sue. She identifies her family as one of the major influences on her values and how she has lived her life.

Her father, James Morrison Ellis (Jim) held values and expectations of women that were shaped by his appreciation of his own mother who had been *an enormously strong woman ... an early school teacher in the bush, going around in a sulky, educating herself and being quite a disciplinarian but well loved by her students*. Jim's father, with his strong bushman's roots, was also very strict and somewhat sexist. His clearly defined views on the appropriate behaviours for men and women valued hard work in the coal mines and on the land for men and left the learning to the womenfolk.

Sue's mother, Ruth Kathleen Cameron, came from Adelaide Scottish/Irish families. Although this heritage also included many very strong women, there was *a sort of softness, a caring for other people* about her. The outbreak of war directed her away from a career as an artist and into the useful role of nursing. Sue identified that while her mother could be very unforgiving in her attitudes, she was also very gregarious and popular. This family line was filled with strong women with large families of children and lots of caring for each other.

Jim Ellis was the first boy from his country school to attend Sydney University. He paid his way with hard jobs at night and held his place alongside the boys from the rich families of Sydney. He graduated as a doctor, but Sue suggests that his original desire had been to be a missionary and his desire to work in other countries and make a contribution can be seen in his work in Vietnam, Timor and Cambodia with the Red Cross and Orthopaedic Outreach.

In following a traditional path for nurses and marrying a doctor, Sue sees that her mother became someone who was thwarted in developing her own talents and, because of this, *was absolutely determined that her two daughters were not to be thwarted in their aspirations*.

Sue's earliest years were spent in the United Kingdom while her father worked and studied at medicine. She was the eldest in the family that would eventually include five children and, once the family returned to Australia and her father established his medical practice, it was a very busy household. Sue describes how her mother provided the sort of home that extended family members always came to stay at when in from the country and her father brought in students from Asian countries.

Sue herself had an important role to play in the household, pulling her weight in assisting with the care of her brothers and sister and indeed acting as her father's medical receptionist for weekend surgeries. This early engagement in responsible activities reflects what Sue sees as a family value: *worldly goods are not something that you experience. You have to earn them. Nothing comes without hard work. You need to be self-sufficient. You need to make your own fires to do your cooking and build your own houses*. On reflection she argues that this emphasis on making a practical contribution influenced her attitude as a student who was more inclined to be involved in activities than diligently swotting.

Starting Out in Social Work

Sue completed her schooling and had no idea what she wanted to do. Her parents, for different reasons, thought social work would be a good idea—her mother had a friend whose daughter was doing social work and her father thought they did useful work clearing patients out of the hospital wards.

Sue herself was unconvinced and her first encounters with psychosocial theory and casework did nothing to convince her. *I wasn't very patient with individual people who just couldn't pull their socks up. This was a value. You had to be self-sufficient.* Sue identifies that her life until then had been *a fairly insular life down the lower north shore of Sydney*.

However, Sue reports her conversion through her introduction to community development with the young Tony Vinson as lecturer. *He turned a light on in my head and I thought that's it; that's what I want to be. I want to be a community worker.* Tony was teaching from the latest practice developments overseas, particularly in the United Kingdom, and sharing with students the latest writings as they became available. Alongside this passion for community work, Sue also developed a love of group work from her studies with Clare Bundey. Her placement opportunities developed this area of practice, innovating service delivery working with families in communities.

Sue graduated with a clear vision of her role as a social worker in developing communities, and in 1969 innocently took a job with Baulkham Hills Shire Council. Neither the councillors nor indeed the Australian Association of Social Workers (AASW) were clear about her role. Sue found no office available, so she ran playgroups from the Town Clerk's office until he could find her a more suitable place. She had to assert her right to work in this style to the AASW, who raised issues about both her qualification and her preparation for the role. As Sue reports, *there was a fair amount of stubbornness associated with, "Well, I'm here and I'm going to give it my best shot"*.

This role was breaking new ground in the provision of professional services that complemented and enabled the work of the community. Sue proudly reports that ultimately they had thousands of volunteers working in programs such as meals on wheels and creating activities that would draw together isolated senior citizens and young mothers in outing groups and playgroups.

Sue learnt some skills in this role that she utilised throughout her career. One set of these related to the management of stakeholders and working with elected officials. She learnt to consult—"sweet talk" in Sue's language—other service providers and to engage actively in the debates about who should be able to access services. She had at least one notorious failure and reports setting up a youth coffee shop that became the preferred hangout of the Parramatta bikie gangs and Gypsy jokers, which became quite a disaster. The police started to use the coffee shop for undercover work and then the bikie battles started and the shop had to be shut down. However, Sue had added to her enviable list of contacts and when Germaine Greer came to Australia and wanted to do a television series about the attitudes of Australian men, Sue was able to introduce her to a bikie gang, who went on her show.

Sue talks of being slow to appreciate the importance of looking after elected officials, although she had always recognised the mandate that they bring to their work.

An unfortunate experience at this point in her career highlights her learning. She reports that her office (and thus ultimately Sue) was responsible for booking the community hall. One day the councillor who was head of the historical society turned up and, when he found another group of people in the hall, had a heart attack on the doorstep. Sue says she nearly lost her job over that double booking, which was seen to have caused the councillor's heart attack.

She worked in this role—the first created by a local council for a community social worker—until on the strength of her reputation the Mayor of Wagga Wagga recruited her. (Sue initially turned down the job but the mayor offered her husband a job too and thus persuaded the team to move.)

So Sue arrived in Wagga Wagga in the seventies with the feminist revolution and the Whitlam government in full flight. She was ideally positioned to implement some of the big thinking of that government and, through establishing a regional delivery structure, was able to channel significant amounts of money into the region. Sue describes writing a submission for money for long day care children's services the day after she had given birth to her daughter. She honed her skills in community work and developed strategies for working in a positive and effective way with communities that are sometimes quite unwelcoming to outsiders.

In these roles, Sue also learnt to set aside the humility she had perceived as embedded in her training as a social worker and to advocate for herself and those for whom she was working. Alongside these skills she also learnt when to back off from the fight and to understand the organisational and policy contexts in which she was operating. Sue sees the growth in her skills through these years as foundational to her development as a chief executive in the future.

Community Worker to Chief Executive

In 1975 Sue moved to the NSW state government, initially in a role supervising students and then as the senior social worker, before finally securing her targeted role as Senior Executive Officer, Community Liaison Bureau, and later Director of Policy Development.

This was an exciting area that laid the ground work for a range of new programs. As Sue describes: *Out of that came housing co-operatives, neighbourhood houses. We set up the basis of what was eventually the HAAC [Home and Community Care] program. We organised with the Commonwealth to do the negotiations which created the SAAP [Supported Accommodation Assistance Program].*

The role expanded Sue's experience in working within a political context but also in career changes that this context can require. A change of minister resulted in a shuffle in departmental roles and Sue became Regional Director, North West Metropolitan Region. While not a shift she had sought, and one that seemed unjust and traumatic in many respects, it moved Sue from community work into operational management and marked a very important transition in her career.

Sue transitioned into her new role using the analytic and operational skills she had developed in her community work. She worked with the strengths of staff groups within the department but also listened intently to the clients and their advocates. Sue was able to harness the energies of the time to achieve some important changes and cites the closing of the Parramatta Girls' Home as one of the most satisfying of these changes. In her community work Sue had become very concerned about the way in which the home was being used to control young women and she saw closing this institution as ensuring that it could not do future harm. In this highly politicised context of NSW community services, Sue developed her thinking about human rights and the importance of decisions being taken in full recognition of the civil rights of groups such as people with a disability, who were going to be impacted.

Having honed her skills in the region and then as acting director of operations, Sue was ready to become a chief executive, but the decision to chase the role of Chief Executive Officer, Department for Community Welfare Services in South Australia meant leaving her (soon to be) husband in Sydney and moving to Adelaide and a new political context. She saw South Australia as an opportunity to take up leadership in a context that was *much cleaner* than New South Wales, with ministers who took their work very seriously. The government's willingness to appoint a woman to this important role impressed Sue and added to her determination to really make a significant contribution.

Sue brought fresh eyes to the South Australian context and directed enhanced professional attention to the issue of child protection. In stepping into the chief executive role, she developed a way of working with the government, and in particular the minister, that gave expression to her appreciation of the democratic structures within which she was mandated and exercised her responsibilities to both implement the minister's policy and give guidance about appropriate strategies.

For seven years Sue worked with changing governments to ensure that the department operated with energy and that welfare services were enhanced. She tackled a number of controversial issues and gave effect to the government's desire to enhance the resources of the not-for-profit sector and avoid having the department step into address so many community problems directly. Sue identifies as a highlight the work she did to mediate between the government and the women's shelters and support them in moving to a mode of operating that was sustainable and consistent with good public sector management principles.

Increasing attention to child protection in South Australia involved directing resources away from other activities in order to have the staff and budgets that became necessary once the child protection profile was raised. These changes were controversial, but Sue was committed to ensuring that the notifications that were pouring into the department were responded to appropriately and professionally. Her leadership shifted priorities and drove the major organisational change required —this ability to focus on major organisational change was to characterise her work as a public sector chief executive. However, Sue emphasises that the determination of what the priorities need to be is a political process and that she saw herself as the agent of the minister. In a democratic context it is the minister who gets elected and is accountable for the overall policy.

Sue's next career move was to become the Chief Executive Officer, Office of Public Sector Reform. Again it was a career move she had not sought, but it reflected the very positive assessment of her capacities by ministers in the government and once again she determined to find an opportunity in it. For Sue it was a very new challenge, a job in which her identity as a social worker was not central to the role. It was also the first job in which her community work model of leadership and teamwork was not going to be very helpful. However, she was able to use one strategy that had stood her in good stead in a number of earlier roles—collecting a talented and loyal team with skills that complemented her own, to work with her. Together they addressed public sector reform until, very late in the term of a government that was about to be thrown out, Sue was appointed Public Service Commissioner.

While she was an active member of the Institute for Public Administration and was appropriately concerned with ethics and proper behaviour in the public sector, she characterises this job as one that she hated, as *all it was was men ringing up all day long saying, "I want a bigger car"*. So, when the opportunity presented she accepted appointment as the Chief Executive of the Department for Correctional Services. This presented her with some of the biggest challenges of her career.

For Sue, being responsible for the imprisonment of fellow citizens was a challenge to everything she stood for. However, as Chief Executive of Families and Community Services she had been responsible for juvenile detention and believed that there was a way in which the system could be run that was consistent with her values.

However, she rapidly ran into a significant conflict with the minister, who was seeking to establish a very punitive regime. For a senior public servant who prided herself on being able to implement government policy this was a very big tension. The government slashed the departmental budget by 25%, insisted that there be no "soft programs" and demanded that prisoners be required to wear orange clothing.

Sue's response was to seek a middle ground. She actually refused to put prisoners in orange clothing and justified this on the basis of the significant cuts to the budget that had left no room for extra spending. In the circumstances the minister did not push the issue but he did push for many other draconian acts. As Sue reports, *when I wanted the Salvation Army to go in at Christmas time he said I was to lock all the prisoners in on Christmas Day so they could reflect on their crimes*. The middle line was to not allow the Salvation Army to visit, but not to lock the doors.

Sue's approach to the role reflected her years in public sector reform and she identifies as a highlight the introduction of a private prison in Mt Gambier. For Sue this was a progressive move, which shook up the power of the prison officers, who *had constant industrial action going on.*

Bravery is one of the key attributes that Sue says she developed in this role.

Following a riot in a maximum security prison the prison officers implemented their own system of punishments, including keeping people locked in cells for 23 hours per day. This breached United Nations guidelines and was well outside their authority. Conflict with the officers reached a point where Sue sought the permission of the premier to stand down the officers if they were not prepared to carry out their duties as directed. The result was that the prison was unstaffed and Sue and a few senior people ran it for three days. This required great courage, but for Sue it was yet another opportunity to implement her community work. She allocated responsibilities and delegated tasks to the prisoners. She was open with the prisoners about their power and her need for them to co-operate: *If you all behave we're going to have a wonderful time. If you misbehave I'm stuffed.*

And the outcome was a success—the prison was run in an orderly manner and staff came back to work but were docked pay without any diminution of the chief executive's authority.

Although it eventually became impossible for Sue to work with a minister whose values were so divergent to her own, she did rediscover an important mode of operating that she had learnt in social work: *You need to speak in the language of the listener.*

At the policy level Sue was very keen to increase the emphasis on rehabilitation, but she and the minister were unable to find a common language through which to communicate about this. She identified a Canadian program that was proving effective in changing behaviour—teaching prisoners to solve problems without punching someone—and was keen to introduce this with ministerial support in South Australia. Her strategic briefing to the presenters when they came to talk with the minister was to talk tough, to emphasise those aspects of the program that were about prisoners doing things differently and being accountable. Talking to the minister in a language that resonated with his values allowed him to see the benefits of the program and agree to its introduction.

Sue's leadership in correctional services was recognised by her winning the Telstra Australian Business Woman of the Year award, but it was again time for Sue to move on and, through a complex process of negotiation with a head-hunting firm, she applied to lead the newly created federal government Centrelink, designed to be a one-stop shop amalgamating the Commonwealth Employment Service and the Department of Social Security. Sue sought assurance that this was a big job, and it was!

Apart from the major Australia-wide public sector restructuring activities involved, the operating budget was \$2.5 billion and the program budget was \$45 billion. Sue's appointment to the role was controversial. Having been selected for her strong public sector management credentials, political questions were asked about her suitability. In the end two competing South Australian Liberal Party premiers vouched for her to the Prime Minister's office and the appointment went ahead.

The Centrelink creation story is one of technical innovation, but even more than that Sue sees it as a story of the creation and cultivation of an organisational culture. The positioning of the citizens in their relationship with this powerful body was going to be crucial to the new organisation. Sue was keen to see the idea of customer service that she had been developing in South Australian correctional services come into this new organisation.

Minister Jocelyn Newman, with whom Sue worked closely, was strongly supportive of the development of a respectful attitude to clients, but this ran somewhat contrary to the broader government view that people were only unemployed because they would not go and get a job. Alongside this model was the Job Network policy failure that was also blamed on Centrelink. Sue argues that this was unfair and that Centrelink was actually a very successful creation.

The decision to move back to South Australia was a response to professional and personal drivers. The creation of the new federal Human Services Department was not one that Sue favoured and, although she could see that much of her work would be picked up in the new department, she did not want to be part of it. At the same time the birth of a second grandchild in Adelaide was imminent and Sue wanted to be an actively involved grandparent. In South Australia there was an opportunity to do some new work drawing together disability and housing organisations and providing some leadership in governmental responses to droughts and emergencies. Her last role was the CE of the South Australian Department for Families and Communities. A change of minister prompted her to consider whether she wanted to continue in this role.

Sue retired from the public service at age 60. This created another opportunity for her, as she commenced a volunteer role with Red Cross. With her characteristic energy and commitment, Sue now serves on six Red Cross committees and this year is chairing the Centenary of Red Cross celebrations. For her this is an extension of her commitment to working with community.

Honours and Awards

In recognition of her contributions, several honours and awards have been conferred on Sue. The most notable are the Order of Australia (AO) in 2004, for service to the development and delivery of community support services, and for contributions to public sector governance, and Telstra Australian Business Woman of the Year 1995. Sue said, *If my father was sitting here I'm sure he'd say, "You're not proud of anything. Be humble"*. Sue was pretty proud when she walked away from Centrelink, received an AO, and the University of South Australia conferred a doctorate on her. However, what makes Sue happiest is something quite small:

I get an inner glow when somebody close to me does well and maybe because I might have just helped or they might have sat here and had a conversation and off they go and they do it. It's those little things that I get the most pleasure out of.

Analysis of Qualities/Character

For any social work professional, Sue's life story and accomplishments may appear exceptional, but those achievements were real and inspirational. To initiate needed changes, social workers may need to learn from her experiences and follow such paths. What are some of the striking qualities that have helped Sue to accomplish what she has achieved so well?

Tough and Strong Women

Sue's early formative years were inevitably influenced by her parental figures. Her life and the career trajectory symbolise the image and the character of "tough and strong" women, which may be traced to her paternal grandmother. In Sue's words, her grandmother was *an enormously strong woman, quite a disciplinarian, tough* and Sue's father had an image in his mind of a very strong woman that was his mother. Sue's father was a very strict disciplinarian too: hard working, austere and believing in and practising self-sufficiency. While studying at Sydney University, he worked all night at an ice factory to pay for his university fees and studied all day—he hardly slept. Sue's mother was soft, full of love, caring for people and always giving, but also a strong woman. On reflection, Sue thinks that she epitomises the two qualities—soft mother and tough father—though among her peers she is known for her strength and toughness. In all her 40 years of career, in all her positions, Sue has demonstrated herself to be strong and tough.

Hunger for Movement and Action

Sue said that because her father had worked so hard, leisure and pleasure were concepts that were very far removed from him. Whether it was in his practice, home or weekends, he was deeply engaged with work and he could not bear anyone sitting idle.

Such an influence has left Sue always hungry for movement and action. She said, *the fact that I can never sit still, I'm always feeling as though I must be doing something, comes from my father*. When young, Sue looked after siblings and did small domestic chores, as her mother was often busy with social activities. After her graduation, Sue assumed several responsible and leadership positions. In those days community development was unheard of, but she took initiative and established or contributed to establishing new programs and services, such as a youth coffee shop, meals on wheels, senior citizen clubs, playgroups, implementing Australian Assistance Plan in regional areas, relief work during floods, creating social work structure in the organisation, housing co-operatives, promoting the concept of social work in councils, and more.

> On the day after I had delivered my baby girl I was dictating a submission for a long day care centre which had to be in Canberra at midday that day because I'd been promised a long day care centre if I could just get the application in.

Over half of her career Sue worked as chief executive of huge public sector organisations, both in state and federal bureaucracies, where she addressed critical and demanding tasks such as meeting budget targets, change management, Centrelink computerisation, negotiations with unions, just to name a few. In addition, she held several honorary positions or memberships in other organisations, institutions and boards. Since retirement, Sue has voluntarily assumed leadership roles in community service and not-for-profit organisations. As though this was not enough, she has cleared up unwanted vegetation around her house, planted over 2000 trees, plans to purchase an electric saw to cut dried trees, and regularly attends art classes. Many people also approach Sue for career advice and to resolve their crisis situations. Sue said, *I was always looking for work at work. There was always something to be done and there was always a new project. There was always a new book. I prefer to be hands on, doing something*. Hunger for movement and action has been the hallmark of Sue's life.

Hard Work and Self-sufficiency

Establishing social work and community development in unknown territory and working as chief executive for more than two decades is not possible without hard work. Of the 23 years of chief executive work, Sue said that Centrelink got her at her best. Further, she added:

> I worked very, very, very hard. You know, I would fly to Townsville and back in a day, hand out awards, negotiate with this one and that one, come back. I travelled Australia everywhere all the time. I was constantly negotiating billions of dollars in contracts and things.

It appears that her movement and action were on all the time. Self-sufficiency is an overriding value that pervades her thoughts and actions.

Big Picture

From the very beginning Sue was a big picture person and she likes to work on bigger picture stuff. During her social work training, Sue just knew, *one on one was not going to be where she would ever be. But she could do bigger stuff.* Her career trajectory shows how she was engaged with the bigger stuff throughout her community work and executive career in a range of public sector organisations. During her early working life she set up a regional delivery and a regional council. As the CE of several public sector organisations, including Centrelink, she shifted priorities, introduced innovative and big changes, and effectively managed changes, which only a big picture person can do. Sue had cultivated the quality of thinking big.

Human Dignity and Worth—Customer Service

Sue's quality of valuing human dignity and worth and creatively translating that through customer service, particularly in Centrelink (now known as Department of Human Services), is a remarkable one. She revolutionalised the operation of customer service in Centrelink.

The way Centrelink employees treat citizens (customers) who come to receive services has significantly altered. Employees have had to change the culture of their practice and learn to treat people with respect and dignity, including the introduction of an open physical layout of the offices.

Inculcation of this principle and quality, and practice of it Sue attributes to a critical incident in her life and social work training. In her teenage years, when Sue assisted her father in his practice as a secretary, she encountered a patient who behaved rudely towards her. Sue reported this incident to her father and said that she was going to be rude back to people like that. Her father's response was, "You must never be rude to anybody, ever, ever". When Sue said she still would, her father fired her from the job and she never worked for him again. Sue recalls, *I think "It doesn't matter what happens around you, you must always be respectful", was one of his mottos.* Contrary to this, Sue admits, *If I didn't respect somebody I wouldn't go out of my way to work on them.* Later in life Sue learnt to be respectful of everybody, even if she didn't like them, and to work on the whole constituency. That critical incident in her teenage combined with social work training and later realisation helped Sue to cultivate deep respect for human dignity and worth, and that has constructively manifested in her range of leadership roles, particularly in Centrelink.

Great Sensitivity to Injustice, Unfairness and Exploitation, Followed by Action with Human Rights Orientation

Sue's practice not only shows her great sensitivity to injustice, unfairness and exploitation, but also some action to address them. This was evident in her observation of how some children had used or exploited their parents' income or assets to buy houses in Sydney and how elderly people were isolated in their homes. Her experience with Parramatta Girls' Home and injustice meted out to innocent girls/victims led to her decision to close the home and still support their cause in different ways. Against the wishes of her husband, she offered a night shelter in her home to a young boy escaping from police. She also observed how a Russian woman was exploited as a slave. Further, she saw and acted to stop second-order punishment imposed by prison officers on prisoners. She was concerned about the human rights of disabled people and students also commented that she was emotionally involved in issues. These examples suggest that Sue did not tolerate any injustice and tried to stop it when it was within her powers to do so.

Continuous Learning and Improvement

Sue's biography and work experience suggest a continuous effort to learn and improve. This is much deeper than continuous professional training offered by the professional bodies, though such training programs are important for social workers. While working, Sue completed a social administration course in which she learned about how organisation worked. While working in local government she found she was very isolated and alone and had to become her own mentor. She learned as much from a bad boss as from a good boss. Sue spent a lot of time on reflecting and learning from her practice to improve. She learned from her bad experiences in councils. Her self-mentoring involved the following:

> I do an awful lot of analysis of what went wrong or what went right or what I could do better. Why did that audience respond to me and that audience didn't? What have I learnt from that experience? It's the result of a curious mind, but I also like to think it's the result of a mind that might have been influenced by the social work course. It's understanding. You are supposed to learn about self-analysis and reflection.

Sue creatively combined the knowledge of community development and how organisations operate and in that she found a *fantastic chief executive* in herself. In addition to these two sources, Sue learned about when to be strategic and to her all these *culminated into a set of skills which she found enormously valuable later on in her life*. In her third joint position between UNSW and the Department of Youth and Community, Sue did not just do the required work, but learned about how the whole department operated, which ultimately helped her to rise to Senior Executive Officer of the Community Liaison Bureau.

For a short period when she assumed the role of Director of Policy Development, Sue said, *I learnt how to get on very well with helping ministers understand the separation of powers and what they could and couldn't do and integrity in government.*

Sue also learnt to balance and work with different people, irrespective of their right- or left-wing affiliation, though she did not like some of the dirty politics.

As a Commissioner of Public Employment she learned about how to deal with pay rises and how to set up classifications systems and gained knowledge about negotiations with industrial commissions and unions.

As Chief Executive of Corrections she learned to manage riots and taught herself to drive out fear. Sue said that, as part of self-learning and improvement, it is important to understand yourself, to realise what you are good at and not good at.

Strong Will and Determination

From the very beginning, throughout her career and life Sue demonstrated strong will and determination. In her very first social work job, when she was questioned about the legitimacy of her social or community worker job, her response was:

> I was sufficiently ornery that I wasn't going to go.
>
> I'm one of the new graduates in this sphere and nobody is acting in this sphere [suggesting that community work was a new sphere at that time]
>
> So there was a fair amount of stubbornness associated with, "Well, I'm here and I'm going to give it my best shot".

Even a description of a mayor, such as, *He was a man who knew his own mind*, by Sue during her early career suggests her character of determination. Although she was appointed as a senior social worker, she knew where her mind was. She said:

> I thought … being the senior social worker was not what I wanted to be. I really wanted to do community work and I really wanted this community liaison job.

She was successful in securing community work.

Based on her work with ministers, Sue believes that *you can make sure that the proper things get done if you hold the line strong enough.*

Bravery, Courage and Driving Out Fear

Sue's different roles and actions, such as achieving 25% targeted budget reduction by making some security guard jobs redundant, confronting the minister in regard to his ideas and suggestions, handling prison riots and running a high-security prison, privatising the prison, aspiring to become a police commissioner, suing the prime minister's speech writer, successfully convincing the Cabinet about refreshing the information technology for the social security system, testify to her qualities of bravery and courage and ability to drive out fear.

Knowing Where to Take a Fight and When to Withdraw

Fighting has been so much a part of Sue's life that to her it means negotiating with forces, taking your energy and putting the battle lines out. According to her, fighting is necessary *if you are doing something new, going into a difficult challenge, to make a difference or make change*. She argues that *nobody ever walks placidly in a forward line having a revolution*.

Alternatively, Sue suggests to *put the strategy out if it's less of a fight ... in the places where you're going to make the most impact and where the resistance of the other end is going to be least*. She advises:

> not to pay a lot of attention to putting your energy where the forces of resistance are huge because they dissipate over time as you make changes in this other place. They can be marginalised or they can come to the party. Now, sometimes they can't be marginalised.

Thus it is important to analyse the forces that are benign and that are dangerous, and *unless the most evil of the influences is your boss you have to deal with it*.

Sue said there was a whole set of extra skills that were not taught at university: insights about when to fight, when to pull back and when to renegotiate and come back came from *being wise*. Being wise about when and when not to fight and withdraw seems to be a quality rooted in her practice wisdom. After six years of retirement, even now Sue thinks of speaking out and protesting on certain issues.

Application of Community Development Principles to Public Sector Organisations/Departments

When Sue assumed the first operational management job, she took all her community development principles and construed the department as community. She analysed the department in terms of different *tribes* and their interactions and insular actions. She also treated the prison as a community and organised the prisoners to operate certain functions when staff were on strike. The synthesis of community development, organisation and administration/management knowledge and its application in her executive role is perhaps Sue's intellectual virtue that needs further research and analysis. By heading large organisations and departments, Sue led significant public sector reforms and created organisational culture that led to innovations. It would be useful to look at how the synthesis of this knowledge operated and how it can be transferred.

Innovative Strategies

When new innovations were introduced in an organisation, Sue combined social work and market principles. These included supporting early adopters, focusing on the positive energy, *not wasting a minute with negative nay sayers, taking on something that people feel needs to be done, and building on little successes*. Sue suggests that *if you add the principle of initial success onto systems theory, onto marketing theory, you get yourself a wonderful way of assessing how you intervene in an organisation.*

Temperament

Sue's non-angry temperament was conducive to her job. She said, *I'm not very good at being angry. I very rarely get angry. That's my mother's influence. She said at all costs, whatever you do, don't let anyone know what your emotions are. Just continue to be happy.*

Sue has seen people panic and create a whirlwind of incompetence and hopelessness when something goes wrong. So when things get tough, she says, *I get very calm, very, very, very calm because I know that the only way you can deal out of a difficult situation is to have everybody working with their best brains.* Sue believes that *the mood of the boss not only affects the whole of the organisation but it affects productivity. It took me a while to work this out. If you're the sort of person that people are frightened of then they won't go near you. Things freeze.*

Sue's temperament went well with her open-door approach.

Approachability—Open Door to Colleagues and Employees

Throughout her community and executive work, most of the time Sue kept her door open to colleagues and employees. Being busy and making yourself available to colleagues is not easy unless you are committed to such an approach. When Sue was the acting director of operations, she saw a lot of closed-door meetings and she became allergic to closed doors. She had her door open to such an extent that some of her colleagues commented that her door was far too wide open. Perhaps one of the remarkable qualities of Sue as a successful and effective chief executive was being readily available and accessible to her colleagues and employees. She said:

> I worked it so that if you add 24-hour turnover on your desk and touch each paper once as a personal efficiency thing, and subsequently do your email only in two one-hour slots a day, in the morning and at night, if you add the efficiency measures in you can actually talk to people because your wisdom and your experience and your understanding of strategy and the way the place is going and the politics of it, it's much better spent talking to people than having them queue up outside your door.
>
> It's liberating to speak to people. So I want people to feel like that but actually your value-add in an organisation is not that you're signing papers but that you're actually inspiring people with your language. And if you have something to say to them which may not be friendly it is better to say it quickly at the time to their faces and resolve it than to hold it up until later and do a formal interview.

Sue tried to create an environment in which people felt fearless to see her and express their ideas.

Recognising and Valuing Colleagues

Sue cherished this great quality of developing a team of like-minded people with complementary knowledge and skills, giving them enough freedom (with boundaries) to work and giving due credit for their work rather than self-seeking. Sue said:

> I brought in some fantastic people. We also got social workers into the new housing estates out at Liverpool and the western suburbs of Sydney. They were very good days and people who worked with me come up to me and say they were the best days of their lives. We knew no boundaries. That was very, very exciting times. I don't take credit for much of that because it was these fabulous, fabulous people that I worked with that I'd recruited. Some of them had been my students in local government.

Similarly, based on her experience at the Office of Public Sector Reform, Sue said, *I recruited a sharp little team around me, with the exception of a handful, I am pretty good at picking good people to work with me... and I have enjoyed working in a complementary space*.

It is important to clearly explain to working teams what is being done and where they are going and then give them freedom to act. Rather than only focusing on rules and reporting, Sue gave responsibility to people and said: *Here's a big job. Go and make it happen. I'm here if you want me to help you*. Under such organisational culture, she suggests allowing the innovation to flourish, with boundaries around it, and that will help people have a great sense of satisfaction. People enjoy working in such organisational culture. Sue's experience suggests that social work knowledge helps to create a good environment for people and lets them innovate with freedom. She said:

> I've always believed in putting people into bigger jobs, bigger roles, than they think they can do and they never let me down because we constrain people so much. The things that I loved were innovation and people feeling fantastic, even doing the difficult jobs.

Taking Control of the Story and Reframing

In life there are situations where you may feel helpless, humiliated and furious. Each person will react to such a situation differently. Unexpectedly and unjustifiably, when Sue was moved from one position to another, she felt utter injustice because such a biased decision was based on her gender, religion and marital status. No official opportunities were given for her to ventilate. Her ventilation was only tears for a couple of days till her daughter consoled her. Sue recalls:

> That was a bad situation where I could have had a nervous breakdown or could have collapsed or could have taken them to court or filed a worker's compensation or I could have sued the minister. I could have done a number of things.

> No, I am going to take control of this story. So I took control of the story and I reframed it. I'm sure I learned that in social work. You reframe and you go into a different pattern.

Sue's construction of a new story was looking into the benefits of what had happened to her. She thought, though humiliating, it was not bad; she was the first woman to assume that position; that was the only job vacant; she perceived it as a fantastic promotion and informed a political party's backbenchers that the ministry had sent her to look after them. As a first real operational job, it was a wonderful gift.

Similarly, when Sue was made head of the Office of Public Sector Reform, much against her choice and liking, she reframed it in terms of assuming that something could be good and turned it around to find an opportunity.

Focus on Positive Energy

> Although it may appear counter to one of the above qualities—respecting people—Sue said that if people are nasty to her, she just cuts them off; they are gone out of her life. It is important to see positive connotations of it. She said that her mother was less tolerant: *If you hurt anybody ... if you were rude to her or anybody else you were cut off forever*, Sue affirmed. *I have that ... if someone is nasty to me, I'm not nasty back. I just cut them off, gone out of my life. I've got too much other energy. I'm not going to do negative energy here. I'm going to go forward.*

The quality of focusing on the positive energy and moving forward was also an important operating strategy for Sue. By focusing on and using positive energy, she was able to isolate negative forces or elements in organisations and introduce needed innovative changes. Her work in Centrelink amply demonstrates this.

Taking Responsibility for Colleagues' Work

As a leader Sue always took responsibility for the work of people who worked for her. She remained accountable for their omissions and commissions.

> I always accept responsibility for things that go wrong. There's very little to be gained by blaming people in front of other people. Sometimes you'd like to. But the buck stops with you and if you've created an environment where somebody makes a really bad mistake you have to say why did they make that mistake? Was it their training? Was it the rules under which they operated? Were they in a bad way? Did they have a bad supervisor? People come to work to do the best they can. They don't actually come to work to make big mistakes. If you create an environment where people are empowered to be the most they can be, the best they can be, then you can feel happy about that and you can feel good. If they make a mistake you say to their faces at the time, "That was silly". And you use it as a guidance thing.

Speak in the Language of the Listener

Drawing on the experience of working with a minister, who she often confronted, Sue suggests it is an important aspect of social work to speak in the language of the listener. However, she admits that both she and the minster failed to do so (at least initially on Sue's part).

Selling Yourself—Be Your Own Advocate

Sue's experience suggests that the quality of selling yourself or being your own advocate is an important one. She said:

> You must learn to speak for yourself because no one else will. You have to be your own advocate. I had to learn to turn everything that I stood for into sets of positive messages to take them with me. I spent a lot of my life learning how to sell, which is why people would say to me, "You'll never be humble." It's directly because I've had to advocate for myself.
>
> We were trained to be a bit too humble in social work … you're so self-effacing, don't let it be me, let you be empowered, all that other stuff, which are very important principles but some of the social workers … if you don't actually add that other set of skills you are a bit in trouble because you get a bit wet.

If there is a need for developing such a quality among social workers, it has implications for what social workers are and how they advocate for themselves and their practice. Perhaps they need to learn to turn everything they stood for into positive messages.

Image Building: Show that You Know What You Are Doing

Heading Centrelink when Sue did was a challenging and complex task, as it involved merging two organisations and creating a new one with a budget of $45 billion and 26,000 employees. In this role it was important for Sue to send the message that she knew what she was doing, though she did not fully know it. She said, *The images that other people have of you are the images you create yourself. So, whatever you do, don't send out any messages that say I have no idea what I'm doing*.

Sue has seen many men quickly putting up their hands when there is a job or opportunity, whether they are capable of doing it or not. On the other hand, women, though very capable, say, "Oh, am I good enough? I don't think so". It is vital to create the image of "I can do it". Sue said,

> So I thought, well, I am going to create an image of myself that implies that I can do something. I'm not going to allow the language of me to diminish me because we do as women.

So I often fall off this log. I'm not always good at it but I try really hard never to say I can't do it because I say to myself, given the right amount of brainpower I can do it.

It's about how you describe yourself and how you think of yourself and what sort of tape you have running in your head. I used to have a tape, "I'm only a social worker". Then I turned it into "Social workers can do anything". It was a very big shift in my head. It's the self-talk that's important … I've had to all my life sell social work in a sense.

So, social workers not only may need to self-talk that "I can do it", but also build that image within and outside and show that you know what you are doing.

Knowing When It Was Time to Go

In about 40 years of work life, Sue held 14 significant positions, moving from one to another, most of the time upwards. In a high level bureaucracy, often people do not stick to positions for a long time and it is usual to see them moving frequently. Sue said that she knew when it was time to go and she left often on a high rather than on a low and for her it was important to leave on a high. It appears that leaving on a high was an important guideline for her, which suggests leaving with self-dignity and respect. In addition, in many instances pull and push factors just matched for Sue, which might have facilitated leaving on a high. She said, *The push and the pull was more about when I chose to leave, not when it was chosen for me to leave. I don't know. You just pick up the vibes and you just know.*

Work and Family Balance

Sue's life and career suggest that work gained more priority in her life than her family. When she accepted a chief executive position in Adelaide, she had to live away from her spouse for about 18 months, compromising with quarterly visits. Sue also was conscious about the time she gave to her daughter and was keen to become a better grandmother. *You can't make sacrifices if you're chief executive. You have to be able to do it full on. If I had my druthers I would have been a better mother. I always say I never really got the balance right to my family side.*
This may also suggest that Sue simply enjoyed her work and career and achieved excellence in whatever she did. This raises questions as to whether achievement in one sphere often occurs with (reasonable) compromises in another sphere.

Community Development, Practice Wisdom

Drawing on the analysis of her practice, the following tips may be identified for social work and/or community practice.

Cover the Bases Everywhere

During her second job at the council, as she was busy looking after the mayor, Sue said she did not work hard at building the relationships with any conservative or wider constituency. *Later on in my life I would have been much more sensible. I would have made sure that I had my bases covered everywhere. It's a pretty sensible community development principle. I just forgot.*

Disrupt the System Constructively Rather Than Disrupt It Negatively

Sue suggests that *once you can see any community or any space that you are working in as a system, then it is better to disrupt the system constructively than disrupt the system negatively.*

Empower and Get People Involved

Sue said that she was not some sort of random person running around doing good works. She believed in empowering people and doing things properly and getting people involved and engaged in doing surveys to find out what was happening.

Don't Talk Negatively About Anybody to Anybody

Sue received a piece of useful advice from a friend, who said that although people hate each other in the community, in the end they will always band together against the outsider. So, do don't talk negatively about anybody to anybody.

Do not Assume that Social Fabric/Network Always Works for All

Newcomers or returning community members are often excluded from networks. It is important to advocate on behalf of such people and build them into the existing/old community structure.

You Will Have to Defend Yourself Because no One Else Will

While negotiating her first job salary, Sue was told that she needed to defend herself because no one else would. She said that message burnt into her head. Further, she adds:

> from that very early stage I had to learn to sell myself for what I was doing, not for self-purposes but for what I was advocating for. I could never assume that anybody else would speak for me. You are the only person who will defend yourself because in the end the pro-voices will be quiet and the anti-voices will be strong. So you have to get your voice to be as strong as the negatives because you're going to have to be prepared to debate that out.

No One Will Rescue You

Emanating from the value of self-sufficiency, Sue believed that no one will rescue you. It is important to learn to speak and to advocate.

Managing up

In the bureaucracy "managing up" (maintaining good rapport with senior officers) is very important, but Sue admitted that as she was too busy, she did not manage up all that well. *I have been accused of not managing up very well in my lifetime. I think probably that's one of my weaknesses. It's too late now.* In hindsight, Sue thinks that she *might have benefited if someone had come and said you had to be nicer to the people upwards. Probably that was my weakness in life.*

Anxiety, Nervousness and Self-doubt

In the face of Sue's extraordinary accomplishments, it may be comforting to aspiring social workers and social work leaders to know that for Sue it was normal to experience relatively anxious and nervous moments and she honestly and humbly admits those moments in her narration.

When Sue appeared for her first social work job interview, she thought she would not get it. When the offer was made to her she was absolutely surprised. She said:

> I suppose shocked is how you feel but then there's a certain "Oh, my God, I've never been employed. I don't know what to do." I didn't know anything. I wasn't unconfident about doing the job. It was, for me, the lack of comfort was how to negotiate into the workplace. Yeah, I suppose it's all I felt at the time.

Later when Sue was asked for ministerial briefings, she went to meetings with some anxiety: *Oh, have I done anything wrong?* While it is normal to experience it, what is important is the ability to acknowledge it and constructively deal with it.

When Sue applied for certain jobs, she was not totally sure that she wanted to apply. These emotional states or qualities are part of normal human nature, but what is crucial is how you overcome them. We believe some of the above qualities should help people to do so.

Conclusion

Sue's life and career undoubtedly form an inspirational story. She considered that as a growing girl she *had a fairly insular life down the lower north shore of Sydney*. She had no sense of what she wanted to be. She had a sheltered life of which politics wasn't a part of her life and she didn't necessarily understand about governments because that wasn't part of her life".

Entirely contrary to that early life, Sue's working life enchantingly and challengingly covered vast vistas from north-shore Sydney to all over Australia, revolving her movements and moments around governments, politicians and politics, and people from local to federal levels—reflecting a strong character, enviable qualities and operating styles, and strategies presented in this chapter.

Chapter 11
What You Know Plays Out in Action—Jill Wilson, AO

A.W. (Bill) Anscombe

Jill Wilson is Professor of social work in the School of Nursing, Midwifery and Social Work at the University of Queensland (UQ). Her particular interests in social work are aged care policy and practice—older people's assets, financial abuse and residential aged care; community care for older people; intellectual disability service models; field education and staff supervision; as well as general social work practice. The university's research website lists 87 publications for Jill—books, journal articles, book chapters and other outputs; 21 grants administered by the university; and 28 past or present Higher Degree students. She has worked as a social worker in the areas of intellectual disability, child protection and ageing. As an academic at UQ she has taught social work practice, leadership and supervision. She was awarded an Order of Australia (AO) in 2004. Jill holds a Bachelor of Social Studies degree, a Master of Social Work and a doctorate degree from UQ. She is a Foundation Fellow of the Australian College of Social Work, a member of the Australian Association of Social Workers (AASW) and has been active in social work accreditation programs across Australia.

Family Background and Childhood

Jill's father returned from the Air Force following the Second World War. Prior to the war he had worked in a bank. Her mother was a teacher who graduated from Teachers' College during the Depression. Jill was born in Rockhampton and had a brother who was three years younger than her. When she was five or six her parents moved to a mixed farm in the Dawson Valley, which was a huge change for all the family. Neither of her parents was from the country and the change included

A.W. (Bill) Anscombe (✉)
Charles Sturt University, Wagga Wagga, Australia
e-mail: BAnscombe@csu.edu.au

M. Pawar et al. (eds.), *Empowering Social Workers*,
DOI 10.1007/978-981-10-3809-9_11

moving from a modern home with electricity and a dishwasher to a house that had no electricity and tank water.

The farm didn't go very well, as her father only knew about farming from books, but he worked hard and tried very hard. It wasn't a disaster, but a combination of a lack of experience and bad droughts created difficulties. There was a one-teacher school in the area that had been closed because the school could not get a qualified teacher. When the local people found out that Jill's mother was a primary school teacher they asked if she would teach and they had the school re-opened. Jill thinks that her mother was prepared to do it because Jill had to go to school. So Jill went to a one-teacher school with her mother while initially her younger brother stayed home with their father on the farm. Jill noted that in those days female teachers did not get paid the same as male teachers. Her mother received 70% of the male wage and she was put off at the Christmas holidays. As a female she didn't get an allowance to pay someone to clean the school and she was supposed to do that. She didn't get anyone to help teach domestic science, as it was assumed that she could do that. Jill says: *so it was right in your face what the position of women was in relationship to employment and how the state saw family units*. It was an introduction to injustice at an early age.

Jill described her eight years at the one-teacher school as:

> odd—when you look back on it you sort of say it's an odd experience—She's Mum till you get to the school gate, then she's Mrs Wilson, then she's Mum when you walk out the school gate. And you can't talk about school really at home. You certainly can't make any complaints. You certainly can't raise any issues. I could talk to Dad about it but he probably quite wisely kept right out of it. So in that context we didn't have the same sort of experience of school that a lot of kids would have.

She described one-teacher schools as different and being *just big families*, with a relatively large group of 20 students distributed across four to six different classes.

She described a happy childhood but one where her parents didn't understand the stress and strain on them. While her parents grew further apart, it had little impact apart from times when things got heated. Jill refused to take sides and, with hindsight, that experience helped her to see clearly that boundaries were important.

Jill passed the scholarship exam at the end of year 8 and went to a girls' school in Rockhampton as a boarder. Her brother later attended the boys' boarding school in Rockhampton. When she was in the second year of boarding school, Jill's parents moved to work for the Northern Territory Administration—a part of the Commonwealth Government. They were working on Indigenous settlements where her father was a farm manager and her mother was the teacher.

Jill did well at school and secured a Commonwealth Scholarship to go to university. In the context of school she pushed herself hard. She had not had the opportunity to learn a musical instrument or do speech and drama or play netball or basketball at Dawson Valley—and wanted to do all that she could. In these areas she described herself as doing *fairly well at all of them—not brilliantly, but competent at all of them*. Her brother could see her from his school but she couldn't walk up and see him. They saw their parents once a year, due to the expense of going to the Territory. To keep two children at boarding schools—notwithstanding the tuition fees from the scholarship exams—was expensive and it was a struggle for her parents. While it was never presented to her by her parents as a difficulty, as a young person Jill was quite aware that there was not much spare money and she didn't ask for much. She said: *Well, we didn't need much really—different sort of world in terms of possessions a person thought they needed to have to be happy.*

University

The family expectation was that Jill and her brother would go on with their education. Jill received a Commonwealth Scholarship. She described her decision making about careers and going into social work:

> So when it came time to choose what I would do, I didn't want to be a teacher. I didn't want to be a nurse. So that meant I had to go to university. I didn't want to go and work in the bank either. All of those things were things that didn't require any more study. How I lit on [social work] has always been a bit of a mystery to me. In part, it's because when I looked at the subjects that you had to do, I thought, "Well, they're interesting." I hadn't done physics and chemistry for senior … So at that point, the courses I could do in Queensland, because there was no university in the Northern Territory then, were arts, law, economics, social work. So, out of that lot, the social work subjects looked more interesting.

She was probably also influenced by her mother who, during the war, had thought about moving away from teaching and working in the defence forces in something that was roughly a social work role. In part it was also just living in Queensland, which she described as a very poor state that didn't have much and didn't spend its money on services.

Jill stayed at the Women's College at UQ for four years. Her 1965 university year intake was the biggest group that had been taken into social work. The course at UQ had started in 1959.

The university was a very conservative place. Women couldn't wear pants on campus and had to wear skirts and stockings and students did not ask too many questions and did what they were told. But from about the end of her second year of the course that whole environment changed, with the Vietnam War and with a whole feeling that this very conservative, protected sort of environment was needing to change. Like many of her colleagues doing social work, she thought this was all exciting and good fun and threw herself into it. She recalls at that time the school leavers who came into social work with her were very bright, competent, predominantly middle-class women who had a strong sense of social justice and a sense that there were things that had to be changed in the world. They were going to do it. She described the times in this way:

> But at that stage it was a real time of change for all of us. We were mostly young adults. Well, we weren't adults then. You weren't an adult till you were 21. But we were entering adulthood with a sort of sense that there was a purpose in life that was a bit bigger than just you. And … it was a time of demonstration. It was a combination of Vietnam on the one

hand and, of course, Joh Bjelke-Petersen's anti–demonstration rules that said you couldn't meet, you couldn't protest, that you couldn't make a fuss about almost anything. We thought that the police force was totally corrupt and that it behaved in really outrageous ways. And that's become much more a matter of public record now than it was then. But we all thought we knew how bad the police were even though they were saying that they weren't. There were good cops but they were not very evident. They certainly weren't running the show.

And I guess the other thing with Vietnam is that you had friends who had got to the age where their numbers came up in the lottery. We thought we saw a lot of injustice in that context. Everybody we knew in engineering would get called up. Nobody we knew in arts would. Now, this might have been total fabrication but this is what we thought. We didn't think it was fair there was conscription but we also didn't think that the allocation in the ballot was fair either. Looking back on it, I don't know how the hell they could have rigged it but that's what we thought.

So uni itself was an interesting time. It was a challenging time. The whole structure of the course was quite different to now. You did subjects for a whole year. You didn't do them just for a semester. You really got involved in it. You didn't have to write endless assignments. You hardly wrote any. You sat six hours of exams at the end of the year on each of them. So I guess what that did serve to deepen the knowledge you had about the topic. And it meant you had to actually learn it as distinct from deconstruct it. And I think that was a big loss that we struggle to replace now in the context of 13 weeks of teaching and students who are only there to pass exams.

We went to uni nine to five—five days a week. And, if we didn't have classes, we were in the library because, if you didn't go to the library, read and take notes, you couldn't get the information any other way … You were at uni. And you were there and you were with your peers. And you did talk to your peers. And you did develop ideas and make plans. It was a much more face-to-face sort of world. I'm not saying students now don't have peers because they do but they don't spend that much time sitting in big groups together. They're on Facebook or on the phone, just one-to-one which I think is a bit of a limitation.

Jill had a Commonwealth Scholarship but didn't get the living allowance as both her parents had wages. Her mother paid her fees at the college. Jill babysat for a couple of families and one family became great friends. They had five children, at that stage, less than five years of age. She would bath the children, give them tea, read them a story, return to college and have dinner and be paid $2 per hour for three hours work per day. It was a regular income and it wasn't perceived as exploitative. This family were an important family to her and she perceived that she had a clear role in their family being between a big sister and a mother. In third year of university she applied for a scholarship from the Western Australia (WA) government. They had cadetships for their mental health services. So three UQ social work students applied for and gained these cadetships, which meant that they were then bonded to the WA government. It meant she had a living allowance and it took some pressure off her parents and gave her more independence.

Her brother had finished year 12 and went to Duntroon and she did not see very much more of him. While he was at Duntroon he was killed in a car accident at age 20.

Social Work Employment

After graduation, Jill went to Perth. She and another former UQ cadet arranged a job-swap so that Jill was working with people with an intellectual disability (the term at the time was "intellectually deficient"), rather than in the psychiatric hospital. Jill remarked:

> So we just swapped. In those days nobody made a fuss as long as we turned up. We swapped. So, in that context, it meant, I mean, my life, my professional life, might have been quite different if I'd ended up in mental health services. But I ended up there with intellectual disability.

At that time people with cognitive impairment in WA were registered. That wasn't meant to be a control issue but it was used to try and identify where the needs were and how services ought to be responding to those needs. The person in charge of the unit called Irabeena was very forward thinking, as he had a son who had cerebral palsy and some cognitive impairment. He had a very clear view that the state ought to take some responsibility and ought to be clear about its level of responsibility. He said to parents, "we'll help you but you look after the kids till they're 18. And then, if you want, we'll put them in group homes, ordinary houses in the suburbs". To the young new graduate social worker, that gave parents some feeling that it was going to be, for some of them, very hard for 18 years but there was a point when their intellectually disabled child would leave home if they wanted.

This manager created an environment where parents felt life was manageable, even though the task was enormous. Jill was the first full-time social worker in the service and with two other part-time social workers was responsible for all of the State. At that time the suite of resources included specialist doctors, psychologists, a residential facility with care staff trained for the role, special schools with the Education Department, workshops run by the Slow Learning Children's Group—which was a not-for-profit parents' organisation—a facility for people with challenging behaviours and another for children who required nursing care, were physically frail and had cognitive impairment. In the days prior to shunts and other medical interventions, children born with hydrocephalus increased the population of children who were quite physically frail.

Irabeena was providing services to families and schools, services to workshops, and was helping develop new services. The unit also was the place where people were diagnosed and where fledgling genetic counselling could be offered. The work was characterised by an attitude of doing whatever needed to be done in the context of the environment, in order to make life better. Jill worked there from 1969 to the end of 1971 and then went to England to work. She considered this the normal life trajectory for a young graduate Australian social worker.

Her first job in the United Kingdom was as a locum at a hospital in Brompton Road for eight weeks, where the work was in surgery, and then to Catholic Housing Aid, where she worked mostly with women and families who were homeless or living in appalling conditions. Subsequently she worked in a local authority social services department in an intake service that developed not long after the Seebohm Report (A committee chaired by Frederic Seebohm was appointed in 1965 "to review the organisation and responsibilities of local authority personal social services in England and Wales, and to consider what changes are desirable to secure an effective family service"). It was a time of change. The service had an intake system that saw people when they first presented and then put them in specialist teams that related to child protection, welfare (which meant aged and disability and poverty), mental health and juvenile justice. Australian social workers had been trained to be generic, but British social workers had specialisations. In this context Australian workers were valued.

Returning to Australia in late 1975, just prior to the Whitlam dismissal, Jill was asked to tutor at UQ and to run student units that aimed to provide innovative placements to pioneer potential areas of employment and to provide enough placements. She became interested in working with the aged and remarked: *older people didn't really get much attention from anybody. They got parked. You look back now, they got parked in aged accommodation or the families looked after them.* She saw a range of older people, with the referrals largely coming from doctors. Some people's families were struggling; some people were living alone and couldn't manage; the behaviour of some was odd, different, challenging; and some older people just took up a lot of the doctors' time and the doctors were saying, "I'm not offering them anything with this. So you see what you can do".

She and the students at the unit were also involved in developing a neighbourhood centre and school aftercare. The centre responded to the community needs, including running bush dances. They worked with families and people with long-term mental health problems. It was generic across the fields of social work, generic in the methods of social work and generic in context—from work in the local school to work with the local aged respite centre.

Jill met her social worker husband, married in 1978, and had four children. She did not have significant breaks of unfunded maternity leave. Having children changed the dynamics—there could be less single-mindedness about what she was doing in the context of work and more concessions had to be made.

Jill described *another whole area of my life which has been with UnitingCare.* The Uniting Church in Australia started in 1977 as an amalgamation of the Methodists, half the Presbyterians in Queensland and the Congregationalists. The various churches that amalgamated had different services in the community. There was a need to consider the governance of the services being offered and a commission was established. As a member of the church, Jill was asked to sit on that commission. She describes it as frustrating, due to having all responsibility but no authority and limited resources. Her interests were in issues of residential aged care and what was happening in that context and in ensuring the empowering of residents.

In 2004 Jill was honoured for her work in UnitingCare with an Order of Australia (AO). Her citation reads: "For service to the community in the development and delivery of new models of care through the social support sector of the Uniting Church in Australia".

In response to a question on models of care in her citation, Jill commented:

> A "model of care" refers to the core principles that underpin practice. A good model of care will focus on the needs of individuals rather than the organisation. In aged care, for example, there's been an over-reliance on clinical models of care in which professionals assess what services clients' need, rather than involving them directly.

Jill developed a particular interest in elder abuse—especially financial abuse. That arose from work at the student units, because she saw older people being *financially ripped off*. This has led to her work on enduring powers of attorney.

At UQ, Jill has progressed from tutor to professor. She has been Head of School for Social Work and currently works predominantly in research, research higher degree supervision, and teaching social work practice. The UQ website indicates that her research areas relate to:

> Supervision; adolescent sexuality and effective service delivery for young women as parents; the impact of legislative changes in relation to substitute decision making on older people; development of communities in aged care facilities; costs of care and methods of service delivery for older people; policy analyses and developing effective programs for young women with high support needs in relation to their menstrual and fertility management. She is Chair of the UnitingCare Board, the service arm of the Uniting Church in Queensland. UnitingCare is the largest non-government provider of community care in Australia … Previously, Jill has been involved in establishing the Red Hill Paddington Community Centre and the Young Parents Program in Brisbane. She has participated in continuing education programs for a wide range of groups including Queensland Teachers' Union, the Department of Family Services and Aboriginal and Islander Affairs, ethnic community workers, Brisbane Youth Service, and Social Work Departments at the Royal Brisbane and Princess Alexandra Hospitals.

Jill is a long-time member of the AASW, has been part of the accrediting panel for social work courses for many years and has been part of the Ethics Panel. She is a past Vice-president of the Queensland branch of the AASW and was a Foundation Fellow of the AASW Australian College of Social Work, where she was recognised with the following:

> Throughout her career of 45 years, her consistent interests have been social work in the contexts of ageing and intellectual disability. She has also taken a particular interest in the preparation of social work students through field education and she has been a consistent contributor to social work education. She has been Chair of a large NGO Board offering health and welfare support services across Queensland.

Analysis of Qualities/Character

Over many years, Jill has shown and drawn upon many personal qualities.

Honesty, Responsibility and Outcomes

Jill has a straightforward and direct approach that is thoughtful and considered: *You've got to be honest about what you can and can't do; you've got to be honest about what you do and you don't do. You've got to be honest with people so I think honesty is important.*

This is exemplified by Jill's description of an incident in England:

> And I still remember [a] surgeon… [who] wanted me to work with this fellow who had cancer. But, as was the case in those days, he hadn't been told he had cancer. It wasn't seen as good for him. Whereas where I came from, I said, "Well, in the context of my training, I think you have to tell him before I can do anything". And he sort of said, "No, no, he'll be terribly upset". And I said, "Well, he's going to be even more upset when he finds out later". And, anyway, we had this toe to toe standoff. And I said, "I won't see him until you tell him. I'll do other work". And so in the end he sort of said, "Well, you know, you colonials. I'll tell him—but it's on your head". And I said, "Well, I don't know that it is". But it did work out and we could move ahead with the issues the fellow was facing.

Linked to this honesty is also a commitment to taking responsibility as a social worker in a way that is holistic:

> I think the other thing is you've got to take responsibility. It's part of being honest but you've got to take responsibility for what's happening here and make decisions about where you can intervene in systems. I mean, a poor social worker in my view, is someone that only sees themselves in the context of being "I am a family therapist in mental health. That's all I do". No, for me, that's not what social work is; that's what family therapists do. But, I think the strength of social work is in its capacity to see the person in context and to make an assessment of where, within the person and the context and the interaction of those two things, the issues and the resources lie. And, I think that's the strength of social work, that's what other disciplines don't have.

Honesty and responsibility are also linked to outcomes:

> The other issue is, in terms of being honest and accountable, being able to say what we're doing. What did we actually do in that situation? What did we hope to achieve? What outcome were you working for and how much did the person know about that outcome? I think, you know, once you get a clear outcome focus you get a clear capacity to describe what it is that you brought to that situation. Social workers are quite often hopeless at it. You'll never have a power base or an influence base with other disciplines in a multi-disciplinary setting unless you can do that … I've been pushing our students on prac for 20 years to know. They have to say "What skills did you use?" and they still struggle.

Jill referred to social work as being more *mixed* with a community orientation and a focus on individuals in their context. Part of the work is to influence people to leave behaviours that are anti-social and adopt behaviour that wouldn't get them into trouble and/or support people in really difficult situations to cope. But equally, this responsibility and outcomes focus required action at community and policy level:

> by the end of that time we'd closed down the housing aid part that we were doing because we'd achieved what people wanted to achieve so that single women weren't being discriminated against anymore in that context. You don't see many services say, "We aim to

do this. We'll do this'... So it was interesting that we managed to do that. I remember they were going to change the Rent Acts because the Rent Acts in England were very much more protective of tenants, even furnished tenants, than anything in Australia. And they wanted to water down the provisions in the Furnished Tenancy Act. So we were lobbying in the House of Commons. And we had prepared a lot of material. The Scottish Nationals were getting up so we were seeing if we could use them for other views. But I was barred from talking to the MPs because it was considered that they wouldn't take kindly to an Australian accent telling them what to do.

In summary, *you've got to have a plan and you've got to be able to articulate it and you've got to be able to justify it.*

Boundaries and Rules

Early in her childhood, Jill recognised the importance of boundaries:

> [Social workers] have got to have a clear sense of who they are as a person and where they stop and start. So, boundaries are really important and recognising how much of yourself you can bring into situations and how much you should definitely leave outside. So that's something that often students have instinctively but they don't necessarily—it's a skill to know when do I talk about the fact that I too have had, been tempted... and when do I keep entirely quiet... So, boundary issues really matter... when it comes to ethical transgressions, they're often around boundaries, one way or the other or an inappropriate use of power.

Understanding the boundaries between the personal reaction and professional interventions figures significantly and frames the way that Jill approaches engagement in difficult situations:

> your first feeling might be "This is awful" but you've got to move from there pretty quickly to exactly what is awful, awful for who, how did it come to be like that, how do people feel about it ... it's like aged care, it doesn't really matter how awful an aged care facility looks, I mean I'm firmly convinced it suits somebody and if you don't find who it suits, you'll run up against big barriers when you try and shift things. Things are the way they are because they suit somebody and you've got to find out who that somebody is and they've got to be an ally in your change efforts and you try and do it in a way that means they don't lose too much. But, you know, it doesn't always work like that. I think the other strong thing from my point of view is that... I'm very focused on a non-violent approach; I'm not a kill them dead type person. I might feel like that sometimes but I'm not ... within a non-violent approach, you stick to the issues, you respect the person, you just don't like what they do. You expect that that person will be reasonable or will see the unreasonableness of their situation if you can hold them to looking at it long enough.

Understanding the boundaries and rules may also result in an occasional challenge to them. She recounted the actions of a friend caught between necessity and rules:

> a mother had been arrested by the police. And she had an eight or nine months old daughter ... they couldn't find anywhere to put her by five o'clock. So J... brought her home. She wasn't supposed to do that but that's what she did. So we then had to go down to the local

store and find stuff to look after this baby and then the next day get it back. I mean, nobody objected to that. It was sort of saying, well, there was nowhere to put her. What on earth did we do? So I think it was much more pragmatic. You do what you need to do. You bend the rules if you need to. And nothing bad happened to that little girl. She got fostered. They found someone for her the next day.

But, equally, she recognises the dangers of breaking procedures:

one of my colleagues that I graduated with and worked in child protection, thought it would be a good idea to get her foster parents together to have a chat about things. She was sacked for doing that … There were risks then. It's not like it was lollipops and rainbows. Especially in the Queensland context. It wasn't that it was "all things possible".

Idealism and Pragmatism

The issues of boundaries and rules leads also to the consideration of idealism and pragmatism (not terms used by Jill). There are numerous examples of work pragmatism and the desire and ability to confront and then change rules and approaches. Social work lives in two worlds—the world of the ideal and the pragmatic world of the present. Jill comments:

I think the sort of mission or goal of social work is so vast and so enormous, you know that to actually feel you've ever achieved it is unlikely. So I think it's more that the sort of goals of social work are so lofty, the standing of social work is so low in the general community that we've set ourselves a very, very big task … so then we get called "bleeding hearts" or you get called "naïve" or we get called, you know, "irresponsible", encouraging bad behaviour, whatever—which is very frustrating. I mean it's frustrating to be caught in that space I think, between seeing what needs there are and not really having enough clout to make it happen.

In considering the realities of social work and the lofty ideals, a number of Jill's comments are illuminating:

I don't remember feeling particularly overwhelmed. I think it's more, as I said; you do what you can do, and what you can't do—you can't do. So I think it's more not allowing yourself to be seduced into thinking you can do everything. You can't …

I think the other truism is that adversity offers advantages, and that when things do look crook, that's when there's often an option to try something new. So I think for our students, it's really sort of encouraging them to see the opportunities … It's people's experiences within context. The context can look like black to some people and white to others.

Courage and Unfinishedness

Social workers need a realistic appreciation of themselves. In response to a question about courage, Jill defined it as:

I think we absolutely need it, but not foolishly courageous. I think people have to be prepared to name issues that they see happening and have an evidence base to support their allegations and have ideas about whatever outcome it could be and how we might get there.

Unfinishedness rather than humility is a term used to describe a characteristic required in students and social workers:

I think the other thing you're looking for in students are people who are not necessarily—"humble" is the wrong word—but people who don't see the world goes around them; people who are able to tolerate people who are quite different to them; not just tolerate but find interesting and respect and wish to learn from. It's a sort of a view of seeing yourself as essentially unfinished—that there's always something more to learn; there's always more to do. So, people who want things tied up too neatly, they worry me.

Authority

For Jill, authority is a *fact of life*. It is largely a neutral concept that can be used for varying purposes. Acknowledging that there have been situations in which she has had formal authority and power (child protection, mental health, students) and others in which she has had authority based on context, she says: *social work has got a lot of power and authority but is often reluctant to use it creatively... we all have authority in some context and we have less authority in others.*

In numerous examples of working with police and mental health authorities and medical practitioners, it seems that Jill was able to skilfully combine both utility with authority and personal power:

I remember being called out one night to see this fellow living in a really grotty room. He was completely... psychotic; let me be a bit more precise. There was no doubt that he had to go to hospital. But the ambulance was there to take him but they wouldn't take him. They said to me, "Well, you get in the back with him because we're not going to drive with him without someone there" ... We got to the mental health hospital and I said to the ambulance, "Well, how am I going to get back in the middle of the night?" And, I mean, eventually they brought me back.

Fairness and Social Justice

Fairness and social justice were issues Jill first noticed in relation to the discrimination that her mother experienced as a teacher in the 1950s, when receiving 70% of the male wage. But childhood also brought exposure to other issues of social justice and fairness:

Woorabinda [an Aboriginal community] wasn't that far from where we were... when I was a kid, things were pretty tough on those government settlements. People had to stay there; they couldn't come and go at will; there were lots of issues... while there was probably quite a big Indigenous population round where I grew up, you didn't see as much of them as you would now, because they weren't going to local schools and they weren't doing things like that.

I guess part of the reason for my parents going up there [Northern Territory] was an interest in what was happening, and a wish to make some sort of contribution in that context… I was very conscious of it.

In discussing the origins of a commitment to social justice and fairness, Jill explains:

I think the social justice stuff comes from that awareness of how unjust policies were, but I think probably much more as an up-swell of rebellion, that we don't accept what Mr Menzies says; that we don't think the world has to be this way. This way puts an unfair burden on some people and gives other people unfair advantages. I don't know that it was particularly what was preached at home. I mean, it was obviously an element of that, and knowing my parents weren't in the least bit bigoted or biased or racist, nor were they particularly well advantaged. They probably could have, but they had made choices in their lives that meant that they didn't have an extravagant lifestyle. That wasn't part of our growing up.

Reflections on the times and the wider events of history intersect with the individual's situation to challenge and change the future:

I think it's a product of the times to the extent that it was a time of revolt. It was a time of not accepting… there were very strong movements, the baby boomers weren't going to tolerate it… we belonged to that cohort. And so why at that particular point in time a whole generation rose up and said "Enough already", I don't know. In part that's probably because financially things were better. There was more money; people had more options; travel was easier; all those sorts of things. Communication was probably better—you probably had a better idea of what was happening.

I think it's also got something to do with growing up in the country. It's very hard to be self-centred in the country. You're surrounded by something that's much bigger than you; you're a small part of this very big thing; and things are going to happen that will have an effect whether you like it or not. The drought will come, and you deal with it. So I think, I think it's a combination of things.

I think for me personally, I'm a child of that time … I think I always have been interested in understanding why things are the way they are.

The commitment to justice and fairness led to roles related to policy and advocacy for senior citizens:

What I learnt about older people and services for older people was that services are very heavily influenced by policy and that the policy context is critical in terms of creating options for older people. So, when older people were being shoved out of their homes by their families because the families could capitalise on the asset, that was really before older people had advance directives or had EPAs [Enduring Powers of Attorney]. All of that shifted dramatically, of course, when the assets of an older person are taken into account and you can't just take them like these people were doing. It was a theft.

The unintended consequence of policy [was] in some cases it forced older people prematurely into a nursing home and then in other cases it kept them longer than they wanted to be in a home. They're policy issues. A lot of families are perfectly well meaning. But we social workers see families on the whole that are not that flash. So you have to keep reminding yourself you're not seeing the typical family about town. But, I mean, sometimes you are. You're seeing families who are stressed but doing their very best. And the reason we're seeing them is because we're trying to mitigate the stress. But I guess the issues for me were the sort of voicelessness of old people; the way in which assumptions were made about them simply because they were old; the perception that they ought to be grateful for whatever they've got; the perception that they were greedy if they hung onto things that other people in the family thought they could find a good use for. All of these dimensions, I suppose, really encouraged you to see older people as people and as products of their time and people with hopes and ambitions, even if they did have dementia and even if they did have quite significant physical or cognitive problems.

So, it was a strong advocacy role. It was a strong support role. It was a risk-taking role—that if older people wanted to take a risk and they understood the risk—then your job was to support them in the risk, not to take the risk away.

That commitment to advocacy has been at a policy level, but also at the individual client level:

we got involved in elder abuse, especially financial abuse… we could see older people being financially ripped off. Here in Queensland, they introduced the EPAs [enduring powers of attorney]. Before that there were just powers of attorney which lapsed, of course, when you lost capacity. And the Queensland government adopted the position that said our legislation will facilitate families to take on this valuable role. And some of us said, "Look, that's fine for some families but there needs to be some mechanism to check on what families are doing because not all families will do the best for residents, for older people". However, we didn't win that fight … But there is an elder abuse prevention unit [EPAU] that was established. It got set up as an effort for recognising the issue for what it was. Although, when EAPU was set up, it was predominantly focusing on physical abuse. Now the biggest single group of abuse is financial abuse.

The advocacy extends to student social workers:

I mean, having worked with the students for a number of years, we never had any disasters—sailing a bit close to the wind sometimes but we never had any disasters. I was certainly encouraging them to stand in the shoes of the other person and imagine what they'd want. It's a starting point. If you stand there and say, "If you were this person, how would you be thinking?" [then say], "Well, what are you going to do about it?"

Conclusion

Jill Wilson has had an extraordinary career in social work. Extraordinarily productive in academic output, she has also combined areas of practice and embraced new and developing areas of practice.

Describing her approach in an interview (Wilson 2004, p. 9), she said:

I think having a holistic approach—having a view of people and services as part of a whole system. Also, social workers are clear about the links between policy and practice. I think I was also able to use social work skills in getting people to work together. Social work has a strong value base which helps this. Social workers are usually able to find a common purpose with other people and act on it in a planned and deliberate way. It helped that through my social work experience I had a sound knowledge of the practice content.

Jill is driven by concepts of social justice and fairness, a combination of idealism and pragmatism, and there is a sense in which she embraces a purpose larger than herself. She says:

> the focus of the Uniting Church is worship, witness and service; and if, in that context, you don't have service, then you're a waste of space … So I think it is about service; it is about involvement with your fellow man; it is about doing it yourself—not expecting someone else to do it.

Reference

Wilson, J. (2004). *Spectrum: A bulletin for graduates, staff, students, field educators and associates of the school of social work and applied human sciences*. Accessed at: file:///D:/Data/Downloads/spectrum15_feb_04%20(1).pdf

Chapter 12
Virtue-Led Social Work Practice

Manohar Pawar, Richard Hugman, Andrew Alexandra and A.W. (Bill) Anscombe

Introduction

The ten biographies presented in this book offer an important opportunity for social work/social welfare/community and social development/human services students, practitioners and educators, and any general reader to look at these professionals' life stories and some of the virtues we have identified and interpreted from those stories. What is the significance of these biographies? What virtues are demonstrated in their practices? What might we learn from them? Do they have any potential to influence ourselves and our practice? They may or may not be exemplary and we are hesitant to call them so, and we leave it to readers to see what they think. However, the subjects' lifelong practice stories speak of their practical wisdom, at least to some extent in some respects.

While reflecting on these biographies and their virtues, we must pose a crucial question: So what? In this concluding chapter we try to address this question by looking at the possibilities and consequences of virtue-led social work practice, some of the common or core virtues identified in the ten biographies, and the potential for virtue-led social work practice in the future.

M. Pawar (✉) · A.W. (Bill) Anscombe
Charles Sturt University, Wagga Wagga, Australia
e-mail: mpawar@csu.edu.au

A.W. (Bill) Anscombe
e-mail: BAnscombe@csu.edu.au

R. Hugman
University of New South Wales, Kensington, Australia
e-mail: r.hugman@unsw.edu.au

A. Alexandra
University of Melbourne, Melbourne, Australia
e-mail: a.alexandra@unimelb.edu.au

M. Pawar et al. (eds.), *Empowering Social Workers*,
DOI 10.1007/978-981-10-3809-9_12

Possibilities and Consequences of Virtue-Led Social Work Practice

Virtue-led practice is not alien to social work and human services. In our view, almost all social workers and related professionals follow some aspects of virtue-led practice, though the degree may differ from one practitioner to another. Our thrust is how to strengthen that aspect. Importantly, virtue-led practice is not an alternative to current ethical frameworks for practice. From a pluralistic ethical framework perspective, virtue-led practice should have its own place in the overall ethical framework for practice (Banks and Gallagher 2009), and it has not yet gained that place. The fact that virtue-led practice is well emphasised in similar professions such as medicine (Gelhaus 2012), nursing and psychiatry (Radden and Sadler 2010; Robertson and Walter 2007), suggests that it is possible and necessary to have that focus and perspective in social work and related human services practice.

Virtue-led practice has good consequences for the self of a practitioner and for others. Focusing on cultivating virtues helps to enhance workers' self-identity, respect for self and others and resilience. This in turn strengthens the drive to deliver better quality services to people and their communities by making appropriate judgements (practice wisdom) in dynamic and unpredictable situations. It helps practitioners to flourish and excel in what they are doing. It has potential to achieve breakthroughs in practice and theory development. It has a modelling effect in terms of its impacts on others. Most importantly, virtue-led social work practice helps to address the major agenda of social work, social change and social transformation.

Common Virtues for Practice

From a comparative reading of the ten biographies presented in Chaps. 2, 3, 4, 5, 6, 7, 8, 9, 10, and 11, we have identified a range of qualities brought to social work and human services by these individuals, which might be considered virtues for practice. As might be expected, and given that how virtues are defined will relate to context and purpose (see discussion in Chap. 1), not all the biographies reveal the same qualities of practice. However, there are sufficient consistencies for us to identify some commonalities that provide the basis for building a picture of social work virtues.

Recognising and Pursuing Social Justice

Social justice is a principle that is widely regarded as a keystone of social work values (IFSW/IASSW 2004; Banks 2012). Therefore it may not be surprising that the ten biographies all express this, although in different ways. For example, all ten subjects tell of being affected by injustices personally, through members of their immediate or extended families or in the communities in which they grew up. These experiences range from the family poverty mentioned by seven, to memories of discrimination and inequalities in their surrounding communities expressed by all ten. These social workers all regard such early experiences as influential in their path towards the profession. Moreover, they also describe their own experiences as influential in their approach to their early practice.

The virtue of justice in classical thought was regarded as a quality of fairness and balance in the way that someone thinks about other people and acts towards them. While such an orientation to their dealings with others is certainly reflected in our biographies, in many instances these social workers also extend this virtue beyond personal conduct, in that their actions are guided by the conviction that they have a role to promote justice in the wider society: *social* justice. (This connection of the value and action is a demonstration of the overarching virtue, practical wisdom, to which we return below).

One of the important distinctions between the modern world and classical times is that contemporary social theory has shown that, in addition to the actions of individuals, social systems and structures create injustices. So for the social workers in this book, a central value of the profession is found in the way in which personal actions challenge those systemic and structural injustices. The ways in which these different individuals encountered and learned about injustices in society were diverse. For some it was their family experience, for others it was through their observations of dissonance between the values set forth in schools, churches and so on and the actions of those who were teaching them. For others it was in the way they were treated in their earlier lives.

These different experiences appear to have produced different forms of response: compare, for example, McMenamin's work in advocacy and campaigning; Ash's use of management roles in NGOs; Vardon's in government service to promote changes in attitudes and practices; and Wilson's focus on research and teaching to create change. Yet in each case these lessons and insights brought them to a common point that is expressed through value statements that can be seen as a shared professional perspective. Indeed, this willingness to act to promote social justice stands out as a virtue that is expressed clearly in all the lives and careers presented in these biographies.

A particular aspect of social justice that is now widely recognised in social workers is that social structures and social relationships are intersected by many divisions. Identity and life opportunities are shaped around issues of socio-economic class, sex and gender, race and ethnicity, sexuality, ability and disability, age and belief (Dominelli 2002); and in Australia, Aboriginality is a very important dimension of these divisions. In each of the narratives presented in Chaps. 2, 3, 4, 5, 6, 7, 8, 9, 10, and 11 a concern with these issues is a major factor in the understanding and commitment shown by each person. While there are clear differences in which forms of social division are particularly identified, these are all social workers whose demonstration of justice is grounded in experience and knowledge about the inequalities of Australian society.

Commitment, Courage and Resilience

Distinguishing between some of the classical Aristotelian virtues, such as courage and tenacity, is not always easy in the modern world. Research in social work and related fields has suggested that these qualities can be seen in the willingness to take risks in the pursuit of what is seen as right, in the sense of "not playing it safe" (such as with career choices) (see, for example, Banks and Gallagher 2009). Among the ten biographies presented in this research, this is evident in accounts of people standing up for what they consider to be right in the face of opposition or even of threat. It is also demonstrated in the commitment and resilience that was necessary for others to take time to develop their skills and knowledge in order to build up their effectiveness in their aspect of social work.

Courage, in the form of standing up to opposition or threat, can be regarded in many ways and to different degrees. The sorts of questioning and resistance to what seemed not to be right in the world in their younger days, as seen in the lives of Ash, Calma, Hall, Miller and Wilson, for example, are all different. Yet they point to the ways in which these individuals developed both the values that challenged what was not right, including the intention to challenge what is not right, and the capacities to take action and to continue to take action through their careers. So the sort of courage and resilience demonstrated by McMenamin in campaigning and advocacy represents one part of a spectrum that also includes at another point the longer-term persistence of someone seeking to make structural changes from within systems. In practice this equally requires the ability to stand up against opposition and to come back tomorrow and do it again, and the day after, and so on. Equally, McMenamin talks of needing the quality of "doggedness", of being able to stay focused on particular objectives over a period of time. This is true in the same way not only of other community activists such as Calma, but also of those who have held management positions in large organisations, such as Ash, Batzias, Gavaghan, Miller and Vardon.

For these reasons, courage can be seen as a virtue that is combined with qualities of commitment and resilience. The evidence from these biographies is that where courage is clearly recognised as such, it is achieved through commitment to values and goals. Conversely, commitment and resilience develop through the less explicit but no less tangible courage of being able to "stick at it", to stay focused and to take the time that is necessary to achieve good outcomes. In this sense courage is remarkable as much for its expression in ordinary, everyday social work as it is for its more public forms.

Compassion

As a virtue, compassion has a somewhat ambiguous standing in social work. Especially within the radical social work tradition, it has been seen as patronising and condescending, implying a sense of moral superiority of practitioners over service users (Ife 2001). Yet according to Nussbaum (2001), this is a misinterpretation of compassion, which she regards as a powerful and positive ethical force when it is grasped appropriately. For Nussbaum it is important to address the difference between compassion and pity. In the philosophical sense, pity here is the vice that represents an excess of feeling towards those who experience oppression and disadvantage. So for Nussbaum, the term pity acquired connotations of patronising and condescension.

In contrast, compassion expresses the virtue of standing alongside someone who is experiencing oppression and disadvantage (this is the "com" element) and being motivated to act by a strong sense of the injustice that they are experiencing (this is the "passion" part). Thus compassion is measured, respectful and committed to the identity and rights of people and communities. The opposite vice in relation to compassion is callousness, which tends not to be seen so much as a problem among social workers, although it can be developed through what is known as "burnout", in which a practitioner's ethical sense becomes compromised by stress or lack of support (see Hugman 2005). Because the social workers whose biographies are presented here have had long and well-regarded careers in the profession, this was unlikely to be evident, but none referred to this as an issue that they had to address in their own practice or their understanding of themselves.

Seven of the ten biographies presented in this volume (Ash, Gavaghan, Hall, Hyde, McMenamin, Miller and Vardon) refer to compassion as a quality that informs their sense of identity as social workers and/or to the way in which they approach their work. Again, we can see that this virtue encompasses very different types of practice and the approaches taken by individuals towards both the issues addressed by social work and the goals that are set. For some it is expressed in a political sensibility, for others through empathy; for some it is both. Nevertheless, whether being seen as politics or empathy, this recognition of oppression and disadvantage in the situation of others informs their commitment to promote social change through their work.

One way in which compassion is addressed in some biographies (Gavaghan, Hyde, McMenamin, Vardon) is in the capacity to listen to people whose lives are very different from one's own and grasp the issues being faced as the basis for developing a commitment to engaging with oppression, disadvantage and injustice. This demonstrates the way in which empathy can inform compassion and avoid the pitfalls of pity. At the same time, to be able to do this through a long career also requires the qualities of commitment and resilience that have been identified above. Compassion is not uncritical emotionality, but rather is the connection of emotions to an intellectual analysis of the issues and problems that social work addresses. It is also inevitably political in that it demands a response that engages in some way with the social structures and systems within which social need is produced. In part the different ways in which individuals then respond conveys something of their personality, but there is also a common thread in that all ten biographies reveal an orientation to engaging with the *social* nature of need while at the same time seeing this as something that can and must be changed.

Respect for Others and Humility

Together with social justice, respect for others is a major principle informing social work ethics world-wide as well as nationally in Australia (IFSW/IASSW 2004; AASW 2010). This principle is also referred to as respect for persons, or respect for humanity. Respect is also a virtue, which is often expressed in a person being respectful in the way that they act towards others.

In practice, respect can be demonstrated in many ways. One that is common across the ten biographies is that of seeking to listen carefully to what others are saying, especially those with whom social workers practice. In this there is an understanding that people who receive social work, whether voluntarily or not, are often people whose voices are silenced in the public sphere. Respect not only sees this but also seeks to create ways to enable people's voices to be heard. This can be within the organisation in which the social workers themselves are based, or it can be wider, in other organisations or in the political processes that affect human services and life more generally.

Another way in which respect is shown is in the emphasis on teamwork and one's own role as a member of a team. The practitioners in this book are people who recognise and value the contributions of others, often putting others ahead of themselves and making sure that those who have made particular contributions are acknowledged (as in the biographies of Ash, Batzias, Calma, Gavaghan, Hyde, Miller and Vardon). While these are all social workers who in some ways and in some places are "in the spotlight", they seek to share it with others. This sort of approach can be seen in efforts to create teams and other collective forms of working, in ensuring that credit is given where it is due, but also in acknowledging one's own limitations.

The latter characteristic, of knowing one's limitations, was expressed in different ways in all ten biographies. It embodies the Socratic idea that wisdom starts with "knowing what you do not know"—to which in a practice-based profession we can add "knowing what you cannot do". This is a form of humility. As with some other virtues (such as compassion, see above) humility can be misunderstood. It does not require a person to be self-effacing or self-denying, but rather that someone is able to see themselves proportionately in relationship to others. So, it is not false modesty, nor is it a lack of confidence. Indeed, none of the ten social workers considered in this volume lack confidence, but by respecting others and seeing themselves as team members their confidence avoids becoming arrogance. This does not mean that when appropriate they will avoid asserting what they think is right or pursuing what is good. Rather, their purpose is not to promote themselves but to serve the interests and needs of others, especially individuals, families, groups, communities and organisations with whom they practice.

Competence

Knowing what you do not know and what you cannot do should not be taken to imply a lack of competence. In these biographies the knowledge and skills of each person are clearly evident. Only four provide an explicit mention of competence or capability as values in themselves (Ash, Calma, Hyde, Vardon). Each makes a statement about the importance of ensuring that one maintains appropriate, up-to-date knowledge and gives value to linking what is known to what can be done. For both Calma and Hyde, intellectual engagement with the issues faced by social work and the practices that it uses is a virtue. Nevertheless, all narratives reveal ways in which competence is valued not only for its concrete effects but also as good in itself—being competent in this sense is like the functional virtues outlined in Chap. 1, in that the good clock is one that keeps time accurately. Similarly, the good social worker is one who takes responsibility for ensuring that they maintain and develop their knowledge and skills relevant to the work in which they are engaged, which is seen in a commitment to continuous learning. Competence and capacity can be seen broadly—in terms of the ability someone has to make use of their knowledge and skills appropriately—as well as more specifically in relation to being able to do a particular thing. As a virtue, competence lies in valuing both these understandings of what it requires and making that a conscious part of who one is as a social worker.

Power, Responsibility and Accountability

As a virtue, responsibility is evident in a person being prepared to be accountable for their actions and the choices they have made. Although only three narratives explicitly identify this quality, all ten demonstrate it in the way in which each person presents their approach to social work as a profession, to people and communities and to their own role in practice. It can be seen in the way that individuals persist with difficult and challenging issues, in the extent to which people make choices about the goals that they pursue, and it can be seen in their preparedness to explain themselves, their values and their commitments and to follow through on the decisions that are made.

Responsibility and accountability are especially important qualities because social workers exercise considerable power in relation to the lives of service users, whether individually or collectively (Hugman 1991). This is not always understood, as power can be exercised in many forms, including through influence based on professional identity, authority over decisions and resources, being able to set agendas for conversations and other ways that are often seen simply as "everyday practice". The responsible practitioner is one who is conscious of this and seeks to use the power that they can exercise in ways that are focused on the needs and interests of people and communities. This can be in direct interactions with them, for example in ensuring that people receive clear explanations about their options ("using plain language"), or that service environments are not degrading. In another way it can be seen in ensuring that the insights of life faced by people and communities are communicated to others who can exercise power through decisions, policy formation and so on. Batzias, Calma, Hall and McMenamin explicitly refer to protest and activism as part of their professional life, while others such as Ash and Vardon suggest a capacity to resist what is wrong as how they sometimes exercise responsibility. Accountability is demonstrated in taking time to ensure that people and communities understand decisions and options, as well as in working relationships that place them at the centre of professionals' attention as opposed to focusing on one's own skills and knowledge, or on abstract ideas, as the central concern of practice.

The relationship between responsibility, accountability and power also connects with the virtues of courage and commitment, as taking responsibility, especially in the exercise of power, can require persistence and resilience, particularly when faced with opposition. The biographies presented in this volume provide many examples, not only of practitioners taking responsibility but also in the courage and commitment that it takes to do this. This is not only seen in relation to activism and resistance, but also in what can be regarded as more "ordinary, everyday" practice that nevertheless seeks to use power accountably and so to be responsible.

Integrity and Practical Wisdom

Often in non-specialist usage ascribing integrity to someone is synonymous with saying that they are a good person. However, summarising the limited literature on virtues in social work and other human service professions, Hugman (2014, p. 81) notes that in professional ethics the idea of integrity tends to be used more specifically to refer to "the integration of the moral character of the person"' and so "to convey a sense of wholeness or completeness". In the biographies presented in Chaps. 2, 3, 4, 5, 6, 7, 8, 9, 10, and 11 we see integration of this kind as each person makes connections between the values that have inspired and informed their commitment to social work and to people, communities and organisations.

Integration of personal values in these narratives takes two forms. The first of these is in expressions of "over-arching" values, such as honesty, truthfulness, seeking not to do any harm ("non-malfeasance"), and also in ideas discussed above such as respectfulness, responsibility and accountability. In other words, when these are combined they produce what these social workers regarded as integrity. So, on this basis, the practitioner with integrity is one who routinely demonstrates these qualities in combination, as opposed to sometimes showing one and sometimes another. As mentioned above, in ordinary speech it is common to hear a person being described as "having integrity" when what the speaker is intending to communicate is that "this is a good person": the notion of integrity becomes a synonym for 'good'. (The statement that a person "is ethical" performs the same function.) For these social workers, integrity means more than this—as well as being a measure of overall ethical standard, it is how we achieve the ethical standards that we set for ourselves.

The other form of integrity that is referred to is summed up by Ash as *joining the dots*, through connecting professional and personal values. In other words, a person with integrity is one whose values are consistent and open. This comes through clearly in all ten biographies. These are all people whose professional and personal values are integrated. Examples of this include those who described how their ethical approach is guided by a religious or spiritual faith, or by political commitments (or both). But integrity does not depend on a particular set of beliefs; it is about all one's values being consistent whatever their basis. Integrity is the mean between, on the one hand, dogmatism—where one is impervious to other points of view, new information, etc.,—and, on the other, inconstancy—where one is blown this way and that by the winds of fashion, other people's opinions, etc. The person with integrity both will hold fast to their views and values in the face of adversity, but also be open to other ways of thinking, prepared to change their mind in the light of relevant new evidence, etc. What someone sees in professional life is as much the "real person" as what would be evident in their private life. The ethical standards of the workplace are not a mask put on for the professional role and then taken off again after hours; nor does the professional role necessitate putting aside deeply held values that can only be expressed in a private context.

Knowing how to create the necessary balance between values in order that they can be integrated in this way is understood in Aristotelian terms as practical wisdom (or "phronesis"). Such a notion points to the way in which virtues are dynamic practices and not simply static qualities. This implies that they can be nurtured and developed and that integrity is the ability to bring other virtues together and hold them in balance, even if that balance is itself dynamic and at times under tension. The biographies provide a rich account of the ways in which these social workers have developed practical wisdom of this kind through their careers. They have done this partly because they have also been able to reflect critically on their actions and their values over time, but also because they have been open to learning from others and from their experiences. In this, practical wisdom is closely related to humility and the willingness to "know what you do not know".

Other Virtues

There is also a range of other values and qualities mentioned in the biographies that may be seen as virtues. In each instance there are one or two people who identify particular examples. This means that it is not possible to suggest a pattern in relation to these virtues as is the case with those discussed above, as they may or may not be relevant other than to specific individuals or to the professional roles that those individuals perform. One such example is that of faith, as mentioned above in relation to practical wisdom. While it can be seen as an underlying influence across half the narratives, such as in relation to the choice of social work as a career, only two people (Ash, Batzias) discussed it more explicitly. For both these social workers this basis to their practice meant that they identified an ethical principle advocated by Sercombe (2010, p. 13), that the central moral responsibility of professionals is to serve, not simply to provide a service. Both Ash and Batzias also link faith to a political awareness of social injustice, which connects them with the statements also made by Calma, Hyde, McMenamin and Miller regarding political values that are sustained by hope.

Batzias and Miller also use the term love, in the sense of making connections between political commitments and compassion. This term is complicated in social work as, like pity, it can imply a condescending or patronising attitude, or have the modern understanding of "charity". It has also been appropriated by the so-called "third way" movement in social policy (Jordan and Jordan 2000) in which it appears as a justification for increasingly punitive ways of responding to long-term need. What is meant here is very different, as these social workers are referring to a strong and passionate commitment to the wellbeing of others and using their knowledge and skills to assist those who are oppressed and disadvantaged. Similarly, Ash, Batzias, Calma and Miller refer to "volunteering" and "generosity", and again these terms need to be understood not as they are commonly used, but as expressions of the willingness to "hang on in there" or to "go the extra yards" for people and communities or for issues that are seen to be requiring the practitioner's involvement.

Gavaghan and Miller both refer to humour as a quality that they consider has enabled them to maintain their commitment to social work and to the wider values that have been identified in these biographies. This is a personal quality that is perhaps more innate than some others, in that while a sense of responsibility can be developed with practice and encouragement, a sense of humour is idiosyncratic. Nevertheless, for those who have this quality it is clearly of help to them in their professional lives.

In six biographies (Batzias, Hall, Hyde, McMenamin, Miller, Vardon) the notion of creativity and resourcefulness is mentioned explicitly in some way. This refers both to finding ways to assist individuals and families directly and to policy, research and/or organisational practice. However, this quality is evident across all ten narratives. Yet what it means is less able to be generalised, as usually it refers to those virtues that are attached to functionality and are expressed specifically in the context of distinct professional roles. So it is a virtue that can be said to be relevant to function (as a virtue of a clock is that it keeps time accurately) but, given the differences of roles, it is less easy to generalise (in the way that all clocks ought to have that functional virtue to be considered a "good" clock).

Virtue-Led Social Work Practice in the Future

In the last 35 years interest in virtue ethics has gradually burgeoned (Snow et al. 2016; Hursthouse 2012) in general and there is a huge potential for virtue-led social work practice in the future. There is also potential to draw on Eastern virtue ethics knowledge base; for example, Chinese ethics (see Hursthouse 2012). The field of virtue ethics is expected to expand in terms of applied virtue ethics, virtues in role ethics and virtue politics (see Hursthouse 2012). Generally, demand for virtue education and awareness is likely to grow in coming years. Towards that end, further conceptual clarity and development of virtue is needed. The way virtue, good life, happy life, wellbeing and flourishing are understood depends upon the way people subjectively interpret it. Thus people's interpretation and evolving meaning-making of virtues is going to be increasingly relevant.

To do justice to pluralistic frameworks in professional ethics education, ethical code-based education needs to be expanded to include virtue-led practice education. It is important to develop a sound balance between deontological and utilitarian perspectives and virtue ethics and ethics of care. As some recent developments such as the intervention of managerialism and the application of market principles appear to have eroded the quality of services and negatively impacted people and their communities, a focus on virtue-led practice may help to address this issue. As a professional practitioner, excelling in what one does should be an important goal and a virtue-led practice approach may help to achieve that goal.

The subject of virtue ethics needs to be expanded beyond the individual, to include and apply to collective entities such as communities, organisations and institutions. These collective entities also have virtues and vices and therefore they also need to identify and cultivate the virtues that will enable them to function well. Virtuous communities and organisations will produce virtuous agents and virtuous agents will contribute to virtuous communities and organisations.

Research related to virtue ethics in social work is minimal (Banks and Gallagher 2009) and our own research on the ten biographies and the analysis of virtues there is just a beginning. A lot more systematic research in virtue ethics needs to be undertaken in social work, to delineate and develop the concept of virtue from pluralistic perspectives and improve and refine the concept we have presented in the first chapter of this book. It is important to research the practice and experiences of excellent social workers, to identify and learn from their virtues and practical wisdom, and pass the lessons learnt on to future generations of professionals.

There are only a handful of specialised social work ethics educators. To provide the highest quality social work ethics education to students and practitioners, those educators need to draw on the expertise of relevant professionals such as philosophers, ethicists, legal practitioners, psychologists and theologians and get themselves well trained.

The current developments in virtue ethics and their relevance need to be reflected in a careful review and updating of the social work ethics curricula. This will also provide virtue-led social work practice education and training to all social work students and related human services professionals. As there is a great disparity in social work ethics curricula and training, professional associations and schools need to play a proactive role in introducing minimum educational standards. Accordingly, good quality training materials and resources need to be developed. The ten biographies presented in this book are one type of resource for future training.

Social workers have a critical role in enhancing the wellbeing of individuals, families and communities. Their path to developing practical wisdom is reflective practice. The more their practice is virtue-led, the more practical wisdom they will acquire. The conscious adoption and adaptation of virtue-led practice approaches will empower them to contribute to promoting wellbeing of individuals, institutions and communities. In doing so, they will also flourish.

References

Australian Association of Social Workers (AASW). (2010). *Code of ethics*. Kingston ACT: AASW.

Banks, S. (2012). *Ethics and values in social work*. Basingstoke: Palgrave Macmillan.

Banks, S., & Gallagher, A. (2009). *Ethics in professional life. Virtues for health and social care*. Houndmills: Palgrave Macmillan.

Dominelli, L. (2002). *Anti-oppressive theory and practice in social work*. Basingstoke: Palgrave Macmillan.

Gelhaus, P. (2012). The desired moral attitude of the physician: (I) empathy. *Medicine, Health Care and Philosophy, 15,* 103–113.

Hugman, R. (1991). *Power in caring professions*. London: Macmillan.

Hugman, R. (2005). *New approaches in ethics for the caring professions*. Basingstoke: Palgrave Macmillan.

Hugman, R. (2014). *A-Z professional ethics*. Basingstoke: Palgrave Macmillan.

Hursthouse, R. (2012). Virtue ethics. In *Stanford encyclopaedia of philosophy*. http://plato.stanford.edu/entries/ethics-virtue/. Accessed 9 September 2016.

Ife, J. (2001). *Rethinking social work*. South Melbourne: Longman.

International Federation of Social Workers/International Association of Schools of Social Work (IFSW/IASSW). (2004). *Ethics in social work: Principles for practice*. Bern: IFSW/IASSW.

Jordan, B., & Jordan, C. (2000). *Social work and the third way: Tough love as social policy*. London: Sage Publications Ltd.

Nussbaum, M. (2001). *Upheavals of thought*. New York: Cambridge University Press.

Radden, J., & Sadler, J. (2010). *The virtuous psychiatrist: Character ethics in psychiatric practice*. Chapter 8. Oxford Scholarship Online.

Robertson, M., & Walter, G. (2007). Overview of psychiatric ethics II: Virtue ethics and the ethics of care. *Australasian Psychiatry, 15*(3), 207–211.

Sercombe, H. (2010). *Youth work ethics*. London: Sage Publications Ltd.

Snow, N. E., Narvaez, D., & Annas, J. (2016). Introduction. In J. Annas, D. Narvaez, & N. E. Snow (Eds.), *Developing the virtues: Integrating perspectives*. New York: Oxford University Press.

Printed by Printforce, the Netherlands